What readers are saying since the original publication of
The 8-Week Cholesterol Cure

"I became aware of *The 8-Week Cholesterol Cure* in 1987 while I was waiting to have bypass surgery following a heart attack. Now, fourteen years later, my original copy is soiled, dog-eared, highlighted, underscored, annotated in the margins, and still in use. I am grateful that [you] continue to digest the pertinent medical research reports and make the results available in language the general public can understand and use."

—Walter F. Eells, 68, West Hartford, Connecticut

"My use of niacin and a commitment to physical activity has made the difference for me. Your book's emphasis on these lifestyle changes and the explanation that [the] liver is . . . the major cholesterol producer have been a lifesaver to me."

—Richard Miller, 71, Camarillo, California

"At age forty-three, I underwent angioplasty with a stent. After reading *The 8-Week Cholesterol Cure*, I changed my lifestyle even more. Now, at age fifty, I enjoy a healthy asymptomatic lifestyle that includes surfing, running, and playing tennis with low cholesterol and other lipid levels."

—Lewis A. Roberts, M.D., Westhampton, New York

"I had my first heart attack in March 1974. It was a massive frontal infarction. I became a faithful yogi and a strict vegetarian, doing my postures and meditating daily. In October 1984, I had my second heart attack. In 1988, when I read your book, I found out how to prevent further heart attacks. I was born in 1915 and am still active physically and mentally. I believe your book has helped me live a good quality of life."

—Albert Shankman, Stratford, Connecticut

"Thank you for sorting and guiding us through the mounds of information on CHD. We have given your book to friends and family who have had heart attacks or whose cholesterol test results have needed improvement."

—Kay Ingle, Ho

"In the fall of 1987, I experienced a cardiac arrest and underwent an emergency triple-bypass operation. On my first postoperative visit to my surgeon [it was] strongly advised that I get your book. It has now been nearly fourteen years since my operation, and I feel fortunate in the knowledge that I have acquired, and am exceedingly grateful for the good health I am experiencing during my eightieth year. Your personal experiences have been inspirational and your research and reporting in your newsletter have been invaluable to me, not only so far as enjoying a heart-healthy diet, but also in helping me to live a happy, healthy, and fulfilling life in my later years."

—Bob Callan, Florissant, Colorado

"After bypass surgery and following a dietician's recommendations, I still could not get my cholesterol to a safe level. By a lucky accident, I found your book. To make a long story short, my total went from 248 to 164 after three months! Thanks!"

—Osborne C. Miller, Lake Mary, Florida

"Bob Kowalski is my favorite expert on the subject of cholesterol and heart disease. Even my cardiologist refers to him. Bob spends more time assimilating the latest scientific information and putting it in more readable, understandable terms than anyone in this subject area and I defer to him whenever I need current information or the latest in breakthrough new methods and techniques."

—Greg Renker, Palm Desert, California

"Approximately twelve years ago, following a mini-stroke and partial loss of vision in one eye, something needed to be done immediately—the culprit, a [blocked] carotid artery. [I] came across your book [and] I have been following your suggestions ever since. My cholesterol, although stubborn, remains under 200 with basic numbers good. I am still flying, able to pass a flight physical, and enjoying life at seventy-nine. This, obviously, is thanks to your book."

—William W. Beard, New Bern, North Carolina

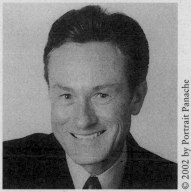

About the Author

ROBERT E. KOWALSKI, a medical journalist for more than twenty-five years, devised this program for his own cholesterol problem when all else failed. By the age of forty-one he had suffered a heart attack and two coronary bypass surgeries, after which he created *The 8-Week Cholesterol Cure* to reduce cholesterol for himself and the many others who have this need.

Also by Robert E. Kowalski

The 8-Week Cholesterol Cure

The 8-Week Cholesterol Cure Cookbook

Cholesterol & Children

The Endocrine Control Diet
(with Calvin Ezrin, M.D.)

8 Steps to a Healthy Heart

The Type 2 Diabetes Diet Book
(with Calvin Ezrin, M.D.)

The Revolutionary Cholesterol Breakthrough

Robert E. Kowalski

the NEW 8-WEEK CHOLESTEROL CURE

The Ultimate Program for Preventing Heart Disease

Foreword by
Jack Sternlieb, M.D.

Quill
An Imprint of HarperCollinsPublishers

A hardcover edition of this book was published in 2002 by HarperCollins Publishers.

HarperCollins books may be purchased for educational, business, or sales promotional use. For information please write: Special Markets Department, HarperCollins Publishers Inc., 10 East 53rd Street, New York, NY 10022.

First Quill edition published 2003.

The Library of Congress has catalogued the hardcover edition as follows:
Kowalski, Robert E.
The new 8-week cholesterol cure : the ultimate program for preventing heart disease / Robert E. Kowalski.—1st ed.
p.   cm.
Includes index.
ISBN 0-06-001132-7
1. Coronary heart disease—Prevention.   2. Hypercholesteremia—
Treatment.   I. Title: New eight-week cholesterol cure.   II. Title.

RC685.C6 K69 2002
616.1'2305—dc21   2001039437

ISBN 0-06-103176-3 (pbk.)

03   04   05   06   07   ❖/RRD   10   9   8   7   6   5   4   3   2   1

I dedicate this book to the people who make my life worth living and fighting for: Dawn, "My Beautiful Young Bride"; Ross, who has matured into a man who fills my now healthy heart with pride; Jenny, my cuddly daughter who has blossomed into a lovely young woman; and my dad, who never had the chance to see my wonderful family.

Acknowledgments

Citing acknowledgments of those who have helped make my books possible has always been a very pleasant task. But this time around I begin with a tear in my eye as I thank the man without whom my entire career as an author might not have been possible. Clyde Taylor, my literary agent at Curtis Brown Ltd., believed in me and my work from the very beginning. After many, many rejections, he finally got my first book published. And in the years since, he was always there for me as our relationship evolved into a deep personal friendship. Clyde passed away just before I finished writing this book. I'll miss him forever.

My posthumous thanks, also, to Dr. Albert Kattus, my cardiologist in the 1980s, who believed in the life-saving potential of my program and wrote the foreword to the original volume.

I'm also very grateful to all the doctors, nurses, and other professionals who have done so much to keep me around so that I could help others fight this killer disease of men and women. Special thanks to my personal physician and friend, Dr. Charles Keenan, and to Dr. Jack Sternlieb, who has monitored my heart health through the years.

Finally, a note of thanks to my weekend golf buddies who supply the friendship, laughs, and terrific memories everyone should have to keep a healthy heart happy as well.

Contents

Foreword

Shortly after I met Bob Kowalski in 1988, I assumed I'd be doing his third coronary bypass surgery. As a heart surgeon who has performed nearly 6000 cardiac operations in my career, I felt certain it was just a matter of time, owing to Bob's medical history. Today I believe that Bob may never need another procedure, and that he has, for all practical purposes, beaten heart disease, the nation's number one killer. Far more important than that, however, I believe Bob has developed a program that can make heart disease largely preventable not only for himself but for everyone who chooses to follow his sterling example and lifestyle regimen.

When I met Bob Kowalski, *The 8-Week Cholesterol Cure* was an international best-seller. I had invited him to do a presentation sponsored by my institution, the Heart Institute of the Desert, just outside Palm Springs, California. We rented out the McCallum Theater for the occasion and were thrilled to find that Bob literally packed the house. When I heard Bob speak, I knew why.

Bob speaks of heart disease not only as an authority but as one who has battled the disease himself. He suffered a heart attack at just 35 years of age, had a triple bypass surgery that same year, 1978, and required another operation, that time a quadruple, in 1984. Couple that with a family history of heart disease, and you can understand why I thought he'd eventually need a third procedure. I underestimated his determination to fight heart disease and the power of his program to do just that.

The audience at the McCallum Theater that night rewarded Bob with a thunderous standing ovation that he thoroughly deserved. Over the years, millions of other men and women have gotten his advice through his books and newsletter. Bob writes as though he's speaking with a good friend or relative in the comfort of one's living room. Warm and friendly, the advice he provides is absolutely solid, based on scientific medical research, not mere opinion or speculation.

Moreover, Bob's program is easy to follow, safe, and totally effective. When he recommends, for example, a dosage of B vitamins to combat the heart disease risk factor known as homocysteine, you can be assured that it will work. That is just one of the many things covered in this newest book that we didn't know about in 1987 when *The 8-Week Cholesterol Cure* was published.

Having spent many an evening in restaurants with Bob, I know for a fact that he loves food. You can be sure that he's not going to be a "scold," telling you to stick with a diet of twigs, leaves, and berries! I don't know of any other heart-healthy diet that actually encourages readers to enjoy steaks, eggs, meatloaf, and desserts, along with their fruits and vegetables. And it works.

Bob's own cholesterol levels stay in a perfect zone, along with all the other measurements important to heart health, including triglycerides, HDLs, and some that many physicians are not even aware of, such as lipoprotein (a) and small, dense lipids.

When people meet Bob, they're amazed. He doesn't look his age, thanks to his diet and exercise regimen. He takes absolute joy in living and he has a passion for sharing his life-saving insights with others. Not only have I gotten to know Bob on the outside, I've become familiar with him on the inside as well. We've done a series of angiograms and other tests on him over the years, confirming that his program really works. Remember that it was just six years following his first bypass surgery that Bob needed a "re-do." That was in 1984. By 1989, he was worried that his condition might be worsening again. Although he felt fine, with no symptoms, Bob was working harder than he'd ever worked in his life, traveling all over the world talking about his books and programs. Was that frantic schedule, which he loved, jeopardizing his heart health?

We agreed that the only way to know for certain was to perform an angiography, an invasive test in which we thread a catheter up into the arteries of the heart to look at the inside. I fully expected that we'd find some blockage, typical of the progression of heart disease seen in the vast majority of patients, but Bob's bypass vessels, five years later, looked as though his bypass surgery had been done the week before. There was no blockage at all.

A couple of years later, we did a technetium stress test. This is a state-of-the-art exercise treadmill test in which a radioactive material (technetium) is injected into the bloodstream. This test shows us how well blood is getting through the arteries to provide oxygen to the heart. Bob not only excelled on the treadmill, lasting far longer than almost any patient his age or younger, but we found that his entire heart muscle was getting a full supply of blood and oxygen. We've repeated that examination on a regular basis over the years and found no blockage at all.

Bob's second angiography was done in 1993. Again, there was absolutely no sign of disease progression. The same was true for Bob's third angiogram in 1999. He has stopped the progression of his disease dead in its tracks, and I have no reason to expect it will ever start up again as long as he continues to follow his own program.

Needless to say, I read all the medical and surgical journals dealing with heart disease. Again and again I've read reports that after about six years or so, patients who have had bypass surgery start having symptoms such as chest pains again. And after about ten years, it's as though they never had the bypass operation, and they need another one. That's because those patients have not done what it takes to stop what is otherwise a chronic, progressive disease.

You've taken the first step toward heart health by picking up this book. Now it's entirely up to you as to whether you'll follow the excellent advice found in its pages. This saved Bob's life, and it can save yours as well.

You *can* fight heart disease and win!

Jack Sternlieb, M.D.
Cardiac Surgeon
Founder, Heart Institute of the Desert
Rancho Mirage, California

Introduction

Suppose you are 41 years old with two preschool children when your doctor says you need surgery that could be fatal, and that if you don't have the operation, it's likely you will die. Pretty scary. The moment I heard that pronouncement my life changed forever.

Well, that was 17 years ago, in 1984. Obviously, I survived the surgery. And I went on to develop a heart-health program described in a book that remained on *The New York Times* best-seller list for more than two years and was published in 24 languages in 35 countries.

The 8-Week Cholesterol Cure came out in April 1987. It seems like only yesterday, but so much has happened since then. Those little kids of mine are now young adults. And my wife, Dawn, and I are thinking about the future and growing old together. Not bad for a guy who might have died young.

But just as my feisty little daughter, Jenny, has grown into a college coed, and my son, Ross, already has his degree, knowledge about heart disease has developed and matured. Over the years, I have chronicled that progress in my publication *The Diet-Heart Newsletter* (see page 255 to subscribe). Yet only a tiny fraction of the population has learned about new information that could literally save their lives.

I never expected to write another book because in 1987 I thought I had all the answers. But nothing stops the search for refined knowledge, and my program has evolved, sometimes subtly and other times radically. Readers who were not aware of my newsletter wrote asking if there was anything new. Anything new? Why, practically everything is new! So my agent, Clyde Taylor, and I began to lobby the publisher to let me do not merely a revision but a total rewrite. Like a zealous missionary, I had a passionate need to share what I'd learned.

So here we are, *The New 8-Week Cholesterol Cure*. To those who read the first book, welcome back. The good news I have for you is that the road to heart health is lots easier today and more completely paved. And for my new readers, there has never been a better time to take the first steps to protecting yourselves from heart disease.

With apologies to those who have heard this tale before, let me go back to the events that led to my unrelenting fight against the nation's number one killer of men and women. Heart disease ultimately takes the lives of nearly half the entire population. Yet with what we know today, this modern plague is largely preventable.

I have a family history of heart disease. In 1969 my dad died of a heart attack at age 57. His mother and sister also succumbed to heart attacks. And his much younger brother had bypass surgery in his fifties. So I rather cavalierly expected an early death and practically boasted that at least I knew what would kill me. But I never thought I'd set the family record for my own encounter with heart disease.

I'll be the first to admit that I did practically everything I could—unknowingly, of course—to speed up the progression of my disease. I smoked, ate fatty foods, almost never exercised, and did nothing to take the edge off personal and professional stress. Suddenly there I was, in Michael Reese Hospital in Chicago, with my heart attack at the tender age of 35. Three months later I had bypass surgery. It was 1978 and, comparatively speaking, cardiologists were still in the Dark Ages.

At the time there was no such thing as cardiac rehabilitation, and no one suggested a program of regular exercise. The diet-cholesterol issue was controversial at best, with most doctors believing it didn't matter much what one ate. When those doctors went to medical conventions, they were even allowed to smoke in meeting rooms.

When the cardiac surgeon discharged me from the hospital he said, "Bob, you're a young man. Let me give you some good advice. You had something wrong and we fixed it. Forget about it and enjoy your life." Not knowing any better, I followed that advice. Six years later, I learned that I needed a second bypass operation.

By that time, I had those two little kids who depended on me. When I was told that there was a high risk of bleeding complications during a "re-do," I had an epiphany. I started to think how Dawn might have to tell the kids, "Daddy went to the hospital to have something fixed, but Daddy won't be coming home," and just lay across the bed and wept. How could I leave Ross and Jenny without a daddy?

Tears turned to anger. Why me? Then that anger turned to resolve.

I made up my mind that I would not only survive the surgery but figure out a way to beat this lousy disease.

In the weeks prior to the bypass, I plunged myself into research. As a medical journalist, trained in both journalism and science, I assigned myself the task of finding out everything I could about heart disease and its risk factors.

At about that time, a medical consensus was developing around the role of cholesterol as a major contributor to clogging of the arteries. So I looked at ways to lower the numbers without drugs and came up with a three-pronged program: a low-fat diet, oat bran and its soluble fiber to remove cholesterol from the blood, and the vitamin niacin to limit the body's own production of cholesterol in the liver. A simple plan, but one that did the job very nicely.

After I recovered from the surgery, I began a structured program of cardiac rehabilitation at Santa Monica Medical Center, following the advice and very strong recommendation of my cardiologist. That led to a long-term regimen of exercise that I still follow today.

Probably the most difficult change for me was controlling my emotions, mood swings, and stress level. But I worked at it as best I could.

Smoking wasn't a problem since I'd given up that lousy habit years before. I know very well how tough it is, having been a two-pack-a-day Marlboro man since college. But as millions of others have shown, it can be done.

It was during one of my workouts at cardiac rehab when a nurse, wearing a big smile, came up to the rowing machine I was on to tell me about my latest cholesterol test. The level of my total cholesterol had plummeted from a dangerous high of 284 to 169 after just eight weeks on my program. Needless to say, I was delighted—euphoric, in fact.

My cardiologist, Dr. Albert Kattus, who is now deceased, shared my enthusiasm. He had originally doubted the potential effectiveness of, as he put it, "cereal and vitamins," but here was the proof. Previous efforts with diet alone had achieved only paltry improvements. And he recognized the many down sides of the cholesterol-reducing drugs then available.

It worked for me, but would it work for others? Dr. Kattus agreed to work with me on a research project there at the hospital. We recruited volunteers, and those men and women, many of whom were health professionals themselves, came in once a week on Monday evenings. We talked about making oat bran muffins, how to still enjoy restaurants, the role of alcohol, the way the body makes its own supply of cholesterol, and how niacin limits the production—all the things I had learned and was putting into practice.

Working on a shoestring budget, I got Quaker Oats to contribute oat bran. Dr. Kattus dug into the remains of a small research budget to buy niacin, which we got wholesale through the hospital pharmacy.

Eight weeks later, as I detailed in the first book, everyone who followed the program vastly improved his or her cholesterol profiles. The idea for *The 8-Week Cholesterol Cure* was born right there in that room.

But in light of more than a decade of research progress, the book has become obsolete. I have kept many of my readers up to date by way of my quarterly publication, *The Diet-Heart Newsletter*. Its existence is mentioned at the very back of the book, but most readers missed it. And it bothered me that they, and millions of others who have in the intervening years become aware of the need for prevention, didn't have a current source of the ways we can all dramatically slash our risk of heart disease, heart attack, and death.

I'm happy to say that time has validated much of what I wrote in that first book. Some originally thought I had exaggerated the value of fiber, in general, and oat bran, in particular. Now the Food and Drug Administration (FDA) allows oats manufacturers to make health claims on packages. Many castigated me for advocating niacin. Today it is recognized as an invaluable tool in fighting not only cholesterol but other risk factors only recently discovered.

I'm particularly pleased when I've been asked to address health professionals at their association meetings, in major hospitals and medical centers, and even at medical schools. Doctors who first criticized the book were soon advocating it for their own patients.

But the most rewarding part has been the never-ending flow of letters from thousands of readers who have written to tell me about their own successes with the program. By golly, it works—and it saves lives!

Now I've had a chance to refine those safe and effective elements of the program, and to supplement them with all that has been scientifically revealed over the years. We know how heart disease develops, what triggers heart attacks, and how we can prevent the disease's progression and even achieve regression.

And it's easier than ever. The mesh of the original net we used to screen out some foods was too small, meaning that we can, in good health, enjoy foods that were previously forbidden. Nuts. Rich caesar salads. An amazing plant substance that can block the body's absorption of cholesterol from foods, allowing us to once more enjoy eggs and shrimp and other cholesterol-rich favorites. New types of incredibly delicious beef have come onto the market.

No more counting fat grams. No more food deprivation. Incredibly, as I gradually eased my own habits and recommendations for readers of my newsletter, some wrote warning that I was treading on thin ice. Weren't all fats bad? Didn't Mr. Pritikin and Dr. Ornish advocate a near-vegetarian diet for anyone wanting to protect his or her heart?

Sadly, advice can turn into dogma. Followers of certain beliefs enter what can only be called cults that allow no progress or change. I am reminded of my mother, a devout Catholic, who just couldn't bring herself to eat meat on Fridays, even after the Church ban had been lifted. Old habits and beliefs die slowly, if at all. And yet, as a medical journalist who continually and voraciously reads the scientific and medical literature, attends as many conferences and meetings as possible, and scours the Internet for the latest and most innovative findings, I'm more than willing to change my recommendations as the evidence demonstrates the need to do so.

I originally wrote that egg yolks were out of my diet forever. Now they are back, and I can enjoy them without guilt. Once I believed that all fat must be restricted. Now I know that some fats are actually good for your heart, while others do absolutely no harm.

Coincidence that I'd been following my own program for all those years? I think not. So what really did the trick? After all, just six years following my first bypass, I needed another one. Sure, surgical techniques improved during that six-year span, but not enough to explain how I could remain free and clear for another decade beyond six years.

Was it the cholesterol improvement? I think that had a lot to do with it. The exercise? Sure. Efforts at stress management? Partly. But I think there was more.

I had begun an extensive dietary supplementation program after the second bypass. It turns out that the very same B vitamins I'd been taking protect against a risk factor in the blood called homocysteine that few had ever heard about in 1984. Antioxidants formed another component of my program. As the years went by, we learned that nutrients, taken in doses higher than one could typically achieve in the diet, protected against heart disease. The niacin I'd been taking to control cholesterol also worked by countering risk factors that have been identified only within the past few years.

And when it comes to the diet itself, it had seemed illogical to me from the very start that one should eliminate the very same foods that had been shown to protect people for centuries. For example, why would anyone tell patients not to eat fatty fish when those who did were healthier? Why not enjoy lean cuts of beef, pork, and poultry when they contain very little saturated fat? Sure, fruits and vegetables are terrific, but they shouldn't crowd out all other foods.

At the same time, I made a conscious effort to increase my intake of fruits and vegetables. And I did so by eating a little of this and a little of that, providing for the greatest level of variety and nutrients beyond vitamins and minerals. Once again, new research explained why such variety is important. It turns out that different fruits and vegetables supply varying amounts of the bioflavonoids, lycopene, resveratrol, and zeaxanthin that we need to protect the heart in different ways.

In medical circles, heart disease is termed "polygenic," meaning that there are many contributing causes. It makes sense, then, that the "cure" should consider a number of approaches incorporated into one complete heart-health program. All that we have learned to this point in time has now been incorporated into this book. I'm here to guide you about all the ways we have now to prevent heart disease.

I've been very lucky during these past years. The shotgun approach I took paid off. Yet I can't help but feel that it's been more than a matter of pure luck. My initial motivation was to be around to raise my children. Then I realized I had to share my knowledge and findings with others. I sometimes jokingly tell my friends that I'm on a mission from God. No, I haven't had any miraculous visions or anything like that. Still, there seems to be a compelling force that drives me on, urging me to continue my personal fight against heart disease.

Most people know what it's like to feel ill with a cold or flu or a more serious disease. And they know how nice it is when that illness passes. But few really understand the true meaning of wellness. That goes beyond not being sick. It's a matter of reveling in one's health, strength, and vigor.

One winter I was skiing with a friend at Lake Tahoe and wound up, by accident, way down at the bottom of the mountain, far away from a chairlift. It was the end of the day and no one was in sight. I had to take off my skis and walk up the mountain to the lodge in my clunky ski boots and heavy clothing, with my skis over my shoulder. My heart was pounding with the exertion. I was soaked in sweat. It took more than half an hour to make the climb. What went through my mind? The exhilarating thought that such exertion could precipitate a heart attack in men my age, but that I was out of danger. I could ask my body to perform extreme exercise without fear. Wow, what a feeling of total freedom!

I recalled that adventure to Dr. Sternlieb 11 years later, in 2000, after my most recent angiogram had been done and once again shown absolutely no progression of disease. Then I asked him the Big Question: At the age of 58, was I still capable of doing that kind of activity without fear of bringing on a heart attack? He told me, simply enough, that I had absolutely no need for any restrictions of any kind. I had beaten heart disease!

For me, wellness is not only a state of body but a state of mind. I revel in my good health. And it's that kind of feeling I want to share with you. There's no doubt in my mind that the program I have developed, and which has evolved over the years, can set you free of the danger of heart disease. You'll feel better than you have in years, perhaps better than you've ever felt in your life. That's real wellness.

The book you are about to read contains the most up-to-date information available. The more closely you follow the recommendations, the better your odds of living a future free of heart disease. Millions of men and women have read my books, and my files are filled with letters from those who now look forward to many years of health and happiness without the fear of heart disease hanging over their heads.

1
Way Beyond Cholesterol

For the past several decades, coronary heart disease (CHD) has been the number one killer of men and women in the United States and in most of the Western world. Doctors have long proclaimed it to be a polygenic disease, that is, a disease that has many causes involving both genetic traits and lifestyle choices. Today the list of contributing factors has grown longer than ever.

At first glance, this may appear to make the situation more complicated. But the good news is that as we identify those risks and learn how to eliminate them, we come to realize that heart disease is largely preventable.

Heart disease begins in childhood. The insidious process of clogging the arteries progresses quietly, and as early as the teenage years, tests can reveal significant blockage. Obviously, the time to begin preventive measures is as soon as possible.

That said, it's never too late to start prevention. By identifying your personal risk factors and dealing with them effectively, you can absolutely and unequivocally stop the progression of disease at any point in the cycle. Assuming that CHD hasn't already developed to the point of putting you at risk of a heart attack or making you a candidate for bypass surgery, you can halt the disease process and perhaps even reverse it before one of these cardiac events occurs. This is called primary prevention. And even if you have already had a heart attack, otherwise known as a myocardial infarction (MI), bypass surgery, or angioplasty, you can still take the measures needed to make sure you stop the progression of the disease. That is called secondary prevention.

Sadly, most people lack either the knowledge or the incentive to take preventive measures to heart. This is true for both primary and secondary prevention. I understand that to some extent: Human nature makes us all feel that "It won't happen to me." But what about those who have already had a run-in with heart disease and continue to live their lives as they always have? To me that's like seeing a car or truck speeding down the street and stepping off the curb anyway.

A growing number of cardiologists and other physicians are becoming advocates of what is termed "aggressive secondary prevention"— that is to say, taking all the steps necessary to not only modify but completely eliminate known risk factors such as elevated cholesterol levels or high blood pressure. My personal hero among those doctors is Sidney Smith, past president of the American Heart Association (AHA) and professor of medicine at the University of North Carolina at Chapel Hill. Dr. Smith, who used his AHA presidency as a pulpit to preach the gospel of aggressive secondary prevention to his peers in cardiology, has done much to change the way doctors treat their patients.

I go a step further. Certainly it's logical to do everything possible to avoid a second heart attack, but why not be just as aggressive in avoiding the first one? That's what this book is all about: aggressive primary, as well as secondary, prevention. Heart disease is the enemy. A ruthless killer. Worse than anything dreamed up in Hollywood horror movies or ancient myths. Now is the time to pick up that sword of aggressive prevention and fight back.

Today we have gone way beyond cholesterol in identifying the many risk factors that contribute to heart disease. For now, we can't do much about changing the genes that make one particularly susceptible to CHD. Maybe someday soon. But by realizing that others in our families have fallen victim, we are forewarned and forearmed. Now let's turn to the risk factors.

CHOLESTEROL: THE GRANDDADDY OF 'EM ALL

Way back in the 1950s, doctors in Framingham, Massachusetts, began a long-term study of that town's male citizens. They did blood tests, measured blood pressure, and watched and waited. Over a period of many years, certain correlations became clearer and clearer. Men who suffered heart attacks were most likely to be those who had elevated cholesterol levels in their blood. That began a controversy that raged for years.

Since the cholesterol measured in the blood, and later found in the blocked arteries of those who had died of heart attacks, was the same as the cholesterol found in animal foods, the logical conclusion was to limit the amount of cholesterol in the diet. But that didn't do much to lower blood cholesterol, and the connection to saturated fat was totally unknown in those days. I could write a whole book on the history of the debate around diet and heart disease, but the conclusion would be the simple fact that we now have proof positive that cholesterol levels in the blood do, in fact, play a major role in developing heart disease. And today we have the means at our disposal to lower cholesterol to harmless levels.

Just for the record, cholesterol is a chemical substance found in all animals, including humans. We all need it and we can't live without it. The body uses cholesterol to manufacture digestive enzymes, a variety of hormones, and the protective sheath around nerves. About 80 percent of the cholesterol found in our bloodstream is made by the body itself, mainly in the liver. Our diet contributes to only 20 percent or less.

That's why dietary measures alone often can't get cholesterol levels down sufficiently, particularly in those individuals with a genetic tendency to produce too much of the stuff. Diet alone typically lowers cholesterol levels by about 6 percent. Extreme dietary restrictions, which few people are willing to make, can lower levels further. But when one combines a reasonably heart-healthy diet with other measures, even the highest cholesterol numbers fall into the healthy zone. More about that as I "spin this yarn" throughout the book.

Why is cholesterol so important? Simply enough, it is an indispensable ingredient in making the gruel that forms blockages, known as plaque, in the arteries. Forget the outdated image of clogged iron plumbing. Instead, plaque is actually formed within the layers of the artery, forming bulges that interfere with blood flow. A bulge is termed an "atheroma," from the Greek, meaning a tumor formed of a gruel of components. The concomitant hardening of the artery is described as "sclerotic." Hence the name of the disease, atherosclerosis.

We're not exactly sure what precipitates plaque formation. It may be an injury to the lining of the artery and the body's subsequent effort to heal the damage. Cutting-edge research today focuses on the inner lining of the arterial wall called the endothelium. The trick, it appears, is to keep that lining pliant and healthy so that it doesn't suffer the injuries that can lead to plaque formation.

We do know that when the endothelium is injured in some way, types of white blood cells called macrophages and monocytes arrive at the site and develop into forms termed "foam cells." Cholesterol gets mixed into the gruel along with other debris. Without that cholesterol, the plaque cannot form. And when cholesterol levels in the blood are high, plaque size increases. Those with low cholesterol counts just don't develop that blockage as efficiently, although, as we'll see, other factors come into play.

A world authority on heart disease, Dr. Lars Wilhelmsen of Gothenburg University in Sweden says that 80 to 90 percent of all heart attacks can be explained by the presence of high cholesterol levels. Other factors come into play for the remaining 10 to 20 percent.

Critics of the cholesterol theory of heart disease once pointed to the fact that those 10 to 20 percent of heart attack victims had "normal" cholesterol levels. But it turns out that what was once considered normal may be average, but it certainly is not healthy for one's heart. Add other risk factors to that average amount of cholesterol circulating in the blood and you have the recipe for heart disease.

We've also learned a whole lot more about differences in plaque. In the past, doctors most feared large blockages that might impede the flow of blood, especially when a large clot might come floating through. Today we know it's actually the newer, smaller plaques that are the most dangerous.

Those so-called vulnerable plaques are filled with a gooey fluid containing the ingredients of the gruel. The tip, or cap, of the plaque is soft and can be easily broken or torn off by sudden exertion or the shear force of blood flowing across it and spill its contents into the bloodstream. That, in turn, precipitates a large clot that can become lodged in a narrowed artery, shutting off blood flow and causing a heart attack. The term "myocardial infarction" refers to the damage, or infarction, done to the heart muscle, or myocardium, when reduced blood supply deprives the muscle of vital oxygen.

As plaques mature, they begin to harden, owing to the deposition of calcium. The larger the plaque, the more calcium. The good news is that the calcium actually stabilizes the plaque, making it less likely to rupture. The bad news is that the large plaque narrows the artery, limiting blood flow to the heart muscle.

Doctors are now using a test procedure called electron-beam computed tomography (EBCT) to detect calcium deposition in coronary arteries. Based on calcium scores, they can determine a person's risk. More about EBCT in "Screening for Calcium in Arteries," below.

But there is a better way to stabilize arterial plaque than waiting for calcium to harden it. Dr. Valentin Fuster at Mount Sinai Medical Center is the pioneering researcher in the field of vulnerable plaques. He says that by lowering cholesterol levels sufficiently one can expect stabilization of plaque, and virtual elimination of heart attack risk, in as little as six months. How's that for incentive?

Cholesterol itself is a waxy, yellowish substance that is insoluble in water. As such, it cannot be transported in the bloodstream. That is the job of a fatty substance called lipoprotein, which combines with cholesterol to facilitate movement through the blood. Picture the lipoprotein-cholesterol combination as a transport system with various forms.

Low-density lipoprotein (LDL) cholesterol, the "bad" kind, transports cholesterol to tissues, including our arteries, for deposit. High-density lipoprotein (HDL) cholesterol, the "good" kind, transports cholesterol away from tissues and back to the liver, where it can be properly disposed of.

An easy way to remember all this is that you want to have high levels of HDL, the "good" cholesterol, and low levels of LDL, the "bad" cholesterol. HDL and LDL together equal one's total cholesterol (TC).

TESTING CHOLESTEROL LEVELS

A government-sponsored agency called the National Cholesterol Education Program (NCEP), in collaboration with the American Heart Association and other medical organizations, has issued guidelines for cholesterol levels, as measured in milligrams per deciliter, or mg/dL. To keep things as simple as possible, I'll simply refer to the number, rather than continuously citing the mg/dL.* The third, most recent revision was published in May 2001. Normal total cholesterol counts are less than 200. Normal LDL cholesterol is less than 130. Borderline high TC is from 200 to 230, with LDL at 130 to 139. The NCEP now recommends that levels of the protective HDL cholesterol be no lower than 40 for men and 45 for women.

Those are the numbers NCEP considers as maximum. But especially for those at high risk, including individuals who have already suffered a cardiac event or who have two or more additional CHD risk factors, the prescribed counts drop to no more than 180 for total cholesterol and less than 100 for LDL.

Looking at the research we find that those at least risk of heart attack have TC counts in the 150 to 160 range. As TC rises from 160 to 180, risk slightly and gradually goes up. After 180, the slope of the risk curve sharply increases. After 200, the curve goes up even more. And after 230, it soars. Similarly, risk owing to LDL is least with

* To convert U.S. cholesterol measurements (TC, LDL, HDL) in mg/dL to metric readings, divide by 38.67 to obtain equivalents in millimoles per liter (mmol/L). To convert triglyceride numbers in mg/dL to mmol/L, divide by 88.5.

counts of 70 to 80. That risk increases only slightly as the number goes from 80 to 100. Then it takes off from 100 to 130, and after 130 the risk is, well, pretty scary.

Now, here's the deal. Do you want to wait until you have a heart attack or need bypass surgery before you get your total cholesterol down under 200 and your LDL under 100? I leave that decision to you. Since my second bypass in 1984, my own TC has been less than 180, with an LDL of about 100 or less. As the research came in demonstrating the superiority of even lower numbers, I brought my TC down to between 150 and 160 and my LDL into a typical range of 70 to 80.

The research I refer to demonstrates the simple fact that as TC and LDL numbers get down into that ideal range, the progression of heart disease is virtually halted and sometimes regression even occurs.

Now, what about that "good" HDL cholesterol? We want it as high as possible. HDL counts for men should be no less than 40 and no less than 45 for women. Again, the higher the better.

HDL counts are most likely genetically determined, but there are some things we can do to get them up higher. First, lose weight if you are overweight. With the approval and supervision of your physician, if you've been sedentary, start doing regular exercise. Moderate alcohol consumption (two drinks per day maximum for men and one for women) tends to raise HDL counts, although no one in his or her right mind would suggest to a current nondrinker to imbibe for the good of his or her heart. More on that on page 94. Smokers have lower HDL counts, so quit.

Studies in 1999 and 2000 have shown the heart protection gained by elevating HDL counts by way of either the prescription drug gemfibrozil (Lopid) or the vitamin niacin. I am a strong advocate of niacin and have devoted an entire chapter to it in this book. And a new supplement called pantethine can raise HDL dramatically.

RISK RATIOS

An even more accurate predictor of heart disease risk than either total cholesterol, LDL, or HDL is the ratio of those numbers. Two ratios have been used: TC to HDL and LDL to HDL. Of the two, the ratio of TC to HDL has been shown to be the better determinant. Let's look at a few specific examples.

Let's say a man has a total cholesterol of 220 and an HDL of 30. The ratio would be 220/30. Thus, dividing 30 into 220 gives us the number 7.33, which is said to be his risk ratio. For men, that number should be no higher than 4.5. So this individual should both lower his TC and attempt to raise his HDL. A healthier example would be a man with a TC of 170 and an HDL of 50. His risk ratio would be 3.4. For women, the risk ratio should be no higher than 4.0. An example of that would be a TC of 200 and an HDL of 50.

Preliminary research indicates that a particularly accurate predictor of CHD risk is what is termed non-HDL cholesterol. The number derived counts all the cholesterol other than HDL, including both the low-density lipoprotein and very-low-density lipoprotein (VLDL) cholesterol.

This makes sense since the HDL is protective, and all other forms of cholesterol, including LDL and VLDL and possible other particles, are deleterious. Moreover, the current determination of LDL is done almost exclusively by a mathematical equation. The calculation to determine LDL is as follows:

$$LDL = (TC - HDL) - triglycerides/5$$

As an example, let's say that your blood test reveals a total cholesterol of 220, with an HDL of 40, and triglycerides at 180. The calculation would be:

$$
\begin{aligned}
LDL &= (220 - 40) - 180/5 \\
&= (220 - 40) - 36 \\
&= 144 \text{ (at risk)}
\end{aligned}
$$

Needless to say, that is not a very exact way of doing a measurement, since the number is greatly affected by the level of one's triglycerides. Direct laboratory measurements are relatively rare, but may be more available in the future.

TRIGLYCERIDES

Triglycerides are a storage form of fat in the blood and are used as energy. Only recently have these blood fats been recognized as an independent risk factor for CHD, especially when the person also has a low HDL count.

In the past, doctors were concerned only when triglycerides went above 500 mg/dL. At that point, the patient would be at risk of pancreatitis, an inflammation of the pancreas, which is a gland that produces digestive enzymes. Pancreatitis can sometimes lead to pancreatic cancer, which is almost always fatal.

During the mid-1990s, however, research by Dr. Antonio Gotto, then at Baylor University in Houston, linked what were previously considered to be normal levels of triglycerides with increased risk of heart disease. As time has gone on, the levels considered to be safe have dropped, first to 250, then to 200, and now most authorities believe triglycerides should be no more than 150.

The risk of developing heart disease and having a heart attack increases directly with rises in triglycerides. While 150 is now viewed as the cutoff point, risk still exists at 100, as demonstrated in a 1998 study that prompted a major editorial in the American Heart Association's official journal, *Circulation*. Getting triglycerides under the 100 mark seems to be the prudent thing to do.

But how? First, if you are overweight, realize that by losing those extra pounds you will decrease triglycerides. Exercise also helps. Conversely, sugars and alcohol raise the levels of blood fat; some individuals are particularly sensitive. Finally, the prescription drug gemfibrozil (Lopid) or the vitamin niacin can be used to lower triglycerides.

In ways that are not totally understood by scientists at this time, triglycerides are somehow connected with HDLs. Often a person with high triglycerides will also have a low HDL reading, a particularly dangerous combination. Moreover, high triglycerides and low HDL can be associated with elevated blood pressures and insulin resistance, which in turn contributes to obesity. Dr. Gerald Reaven of Stanford identified this combination of factors as syndrome X.

I'll go into more detail in the appropriate section, but suffice it to say now that all aspects of the deadly quartet of conditions in syndrome X respond to the same changes in lifestyle—significantly more exercise, weight control, and reduced sugars and alcohol. Perversely, the low-fat, high-carbohydrate diet so often recommended for heart health can be hurtful to patients with syndrome X because it lowers HDL and raises triglycerides while making insulin resistance even worse.

The best dietary approach for syndrome X is one rich in fruits and vegetables, lean meats and poultry, an abundance of fish, especially the fatty varieties, low-fat and nonfat dairy foods, whole-grain cereals, and a rather liberal use of healthful oils, including olive oil, canola oil, and so forth. Nuts would be a better snack than pretzels. Yes, thinking has definitely changed since the 1980s!

TAKING THE TEST

Cholesterol and triglycerides, along with more arcane blood fats, are collectively referred to as lipids. A complete test of those fats is called a lipid profile. Every single man and woman, and boys and girls with a family history of heart disease, should have a complete lipid profile done. Commonly this is simply called a cholesterol test and is performed in a physician's office after an overnight, 12- to 14-hour fast. Testing requires blood drawn from a vein in the arm. Fasting is necessary to get an accurate triglyceride reading. On the other hand, food does not affect either the total or HDL cholesterol measurement. And remember that the laboratory will need a triglyceride count to calculate one's LDL value.

Finger-stick testing done to screen populations at such sites as shopping malls decreased in popularity following a peak in the late 1980s and early 1990s. First, early equipment was only able to test for total cholesterol. Second, accuracy was often questionable. Jostling the machines around while transporting them from site to site threw off calibrations.

Improved technology, however, could renew interest in finger-stick testing away from the doctor's office or hospital setting. The Cholestech Corporation has developed equipment that uses a single drop of blood. Total cholesterol, HDL, triglycerides, glucose (blood sugar), and even a liver function enzyme can be measured. And the accuracy of such tests has proven to be as good as those using venipuncture, that is, blood drawn from a vein.

Cholestech takes testing a step further. You can now register at the company's Web site, WellCheck.com, to receive specific advice based on your test values at the time of the exam and on a continuing basis. To find out when testing will be done in your area, check the WellCheck.com Web site. You'll also find it to be an authoritative source of information.

If your lipid profile is completely normal, there's no need to retest for at least a year, and some would say as much as five years. If the numbers show there's room for improvement, you're holding the correct book in your hands to help make those improvements. As you begin to modify your lifestyle in terms of diet and exercise and take either the supplements I recommend or the drugs your doctor prescribes, you will want to repeat the testing about every two months.

Once your profile is heart-healthy, you'll want to check it at least yearly. I personally have a test done every few months, just to be certain I'm still on the right track.

Various factors can influence lipid measurements. If you've been indulging in a little more alcohol or sugary treats, triglycerides might very well go up. Lack of exercise can drag HDL counts down. Moreover, there are normal fluctuations from day to day and week to week. It's very possible to get a reading of 190 for total cholesterol one day, and 180 or 200 the next day. Emotional stress, a woman's menstrual cycle, a cold, or the flu can make a big difference.

Just like kids in school, some people actually "cheat" on their cholesterol test! To get a good score they'll eat all the right foods and avoid excesses for a week before the exam. Afterward, they might go out and celebrate with a doughnut or Big Mac. They're only fooling— and cheating—themselves.

Along similar lines, I've been concerned for some time about men and women who are lulled into a false sense of complacency because their cholesterol tests are "just fine" when they are taking one of the newer, more potent cholesterol-lowering statin drugs, even though their fat intake remains high.

One man I know took Lipitor (atorvastatin) following his heart attack. For months he followed a low-fat diet. The numbers were good every time he went to the doctor's office for a test. So he "experimented" with a Saturday night splurge, eating whatever he wanted. The tests were still good, so he tried two nights a week, then more. Now he pays no attention to his diet at all, and his cholesterol count stays in the healthy range. Is he safe? Research demonstrates anything but.

An unusually heavy, fatty meal may cause a fourfold increase in the risk of heart attack. When doctors at Boston's Brigham and Women's Hospital questioned 2000 men and women about what they had eaten before their heart attacks, they found that many had had a big meal just hours before.

Why does risk go up after heavy meals? Blood pressure increases, blood has a greater tendency to form clots at that time, and a rise in insulin levels can damage the endothelium.

In another study, Tufts University researchers learned that as amounts of trans fatty acids (formed from hydrogenated oils) increased and the levels of polyunsaturated fats decreased, the levels of triglycerides in the blood rose for four hours after a meal. Similar increases in blood triglycerides follow meals heavy in saturated fats.

I've seen samples of blood from people who have eaten fatty meals in the hours just before a cholesterol-triglyceride test. It's pretty disgusting. The blood is actually creamy, filled with fat—not something you or I would want to have flowing through our arteries.

Many health authorities are now talking about the potential for doing postprandial (after meals) blood tests. Such analysis might be far more revealing of CHD and heart attack risk.

Returning readers might notice that I have omitted the charts I published in the past listing cholesterol and triglyceride levels for men and women by age and percentage of the population. With what we know today, such charts are really useless. All you need to remember, man or woman, is that you want your total cholesterol 180 or less, your LDL 100 or less, your HDL higher than 40 for a man and higher than 45 for a woman, and your triglycerides under 150. This is a simple strategy for heart protection, and those targets can be attained within a mere eight weeks of following the program detailed in this book.

At the time of this writing, doctors at the Cleveland Clinic have been working on a new-fangled cholesterol test. A painless, three-minute skin test to detect undiagnosed CHD, it consists of putting a few drops of liquid on the fleshy part of the palm near the base of the thumb. Color changes are measured by a special metering device. The test determines not the cholesterol in the blood but rather the cholesterol that is deposited in the outer layer of the skin. Patients with previously diagnosed heart disease have been shown to have more cholesterol in the skin. Thus the skin test might be used to screen for those with cholesterol-filled plaque in their arteries.

Physicians at San Diego State University have been testing levels of chemicals called "sphingolipids" as another screen for heart disease. It appears that the heart muscle produces those sphingolipids when it isn't getting enough oxygen, owing to blockage of the coronary arteries. Thus, if the sphingolipids are detected in a blood test, a red flag goes up, signaling the presence of atherosclerosis.

Magnetic resonance imaging (MRI) has long been used to screen for cancer and spinal problems. Now it appears that MRI can be a valuable tool in detecting CHD. Refinements in MRI technology now allow visualization of the arterial wall as well as the artery's cavity or lumen. This noninvasive testing can provide information for doctors to make clinical judgments about treatment.

In a study presented at the 2000 American Heart Association meeting, researchers at the Mount Sinai School of Medicine in New York used MRI to find that significant cholesterol reduction led to reduction in the buildup of plaque in diseased arteries. Yes, CHD can be reversed. MRI can be expected to play a more active role in testing in the future, but equipment cost will always be a limitation.

SCREENING FOR CALCIUM IN ARTERIES

You've probably heard radio advertisements for a test said to detect the presence of heart disease by measuring the calcium buildup in your coronary arteries. The use of electron-beam computed tomography (EBCT), also known as ultrafast CT scans, remains controversial, but only in terms of when and where it makes a valuable contribution to the diagnosis of CHD. Should the average man or woman pay more than $300 for such a test? EBCT is not covered by most insurance plans unless specifically ordered by a physician.

EBCT detects levels of calcium in the arteries of the heart. Calcium signals the buildup of arterial plaque. Older, larger blockages have more calcium than new plaque formations. Thus EBCT can only detect plaque that already has calcium.

Perversely, as we have seen, it is the soft, "vulnerable" plaque that is far more dangerous than older, stabilized plaque filled with calcium. Such vulnerable plaque is prone to rupture, spilling out their sticky, gooey contents into the bloodstream and leading to clot formation that can precipitate a heart attack.

Some say that EBCT can be used to screen the general population and detect men and women who are at risk but have not been diagnosed. Such individuals should receive more aggressive treatment, including cholesterol and blood pressure reduction. Other doctors think using EBCT as a screening tool is overkill, believing that it's just as efficient, or even more so, to simply check established risk factors.

However, the usefulness of EBCT in tracking progression or regression of disease becomes clearer each year. Doctors at Harbor-UCLA Medical Center in Los Angeles reported that EBCT accurately predicted CHD progression by measuring changes in calcium over time. Such progression in turn correlated with risk of cardiac events, including heart attack or need for bypass surgery.

Physicians in Munich, Germany, found that EBCT could be used to decide which patients were truly in need of further invasive testing. Some did not need angiography as revealed by a relative lack of calcium deposition.

And at the University of Chicago, EBCT detected women with heart disease who would have been overlooked by reliance on more well-established risk factor measurements. Dr. Joan Briller feels that such testing would be particularly valuable for postmenopausal women with other risk factors.

A CLOSER LOOK AT CHOLESTEROL

While LDL cholesterol is the bad kind that leads to arterial blockage, there are two types of LDL that are particularly deadly. When

LDL in the bloodstream becomes oxidized through exposure to very reactive oxygen molecules called free radicals, that oxidized LDL has more potential for causing trouble. We have good evidence, however, that we can prevent such oxidation by use of antioxidant supplements such as vitamins E and C. This is discussed in more detail in Chapter 5.

In a cruel twist of fate, some men and women are more likely to have their LDL cholesterol take the form of small, dense particles. Yup, that small, dense LDL does lots more damage to the arteries than larger, more buoyant particles. But, once again, there's something we can do about that. Niacin is known to convert small, dense LDL particles to larger, more buoyant forms, thus greatly reducing CHD risk.

Niacin also comes into play for combating a nasty variant of LDL cholesterol termed "lipoprotein (a)," or Lp(a) for short. Doctors pronounce that "el-pee-little-a" and it has been shown to be an independent risk factor for CHD. That is to say, even if LDL levels are more or less normal, and when other risk factors are calculated out of the picture, Lp(a) can be responsible for clogging the arteries.

Levels of Lp(a) are largely genetically determined. Some people are just born with the wrong genes. Diet has little or no impact on Lp(a), nor do the cholesterol-lowering prescription drugs. Only niacin has any effect and, indeed, can produce a very nice Lp(a) reduction.

Should you be tested for Lp(a)? If you have a strong family history for CHD even though you and your afflicted family members have relatively normal lipid panels, it's certainly worth taking a look at Lp(a). That's particularly true if you have had a cardiac event. Again, I want you to take as aggressive a stance as possible to prevent future problems. Leave no stone unturned.

You can have your Lp(a) tested at the same time you get the standard lipid profile done. Ideally, you'd like to see Lp(a) at no more than 20 mg/dL; levels of 30 or more put one at distinct risk.

It appears that hormone replacement therapy (HRT) in postmenopausal women has a fringe benefit—it lowers Lp(a). But unless you're a postmenopausal woman, the only Lp(a) therapy remains niacin. By all means, speak with your doctor about this.

The next two risk factors are uric acid and glucose levels. These were not considered serious CHD risk factors until 2000, though there were earlier hints. They show up when your doctor does a complete blood chemistry test. If you haven't had one done lately, get an evaluation at the same time you get your lipid panel.

URIC ACID

Uric acid is a metabolic end product formed during the digestion of food. Measured in milligrams per deciliter, it is present in everyone's blood. The normal range is between 2.6 and 7.2. High levels of uric acid can lead to bouts of gout, a painful form of arthritis. And now we know that increased uric acid levels are independently and significantly associated with risk of cardiovascular mortality.

That insight into the mystery of heart disease came from a long-term study extending from 1971 into the 1990s done by the National Center for Health Statistics. Nearly 6000 men and women aged 25 to 74 years were followed for more than 16 years. During that time, 1593 deaths occurred; 731 (about 46 percent) were due to heart disease. Deaths in both men and women, black and white, were linked to high uric acid levels, which increased risk by 9 percent in men and 26 percent in women.

Fortunately, your doctor can prescribe a drug that very effectively lowers uric acid in the blood. The drug, allopurinol, has been used for years to treat gout.

GLUCOSE

Levels of glucose in the blood reflect the body's ability to transport this sugar into the cells where it is used as fuel. If the body doesn't use glucose properly, the sugar shows up both in the blood and in the urine. Normal levels are from 70 to 105 mg/dL. A level of 126 or more indicates that the patient has diabetes. We'll talk about that disease as an independent risk of heart disease shortly.

Surprisingly, low levels of glucose have been associated with heart disease as well. Doctors in Texas found that men and women with glucose counts lower than 70 were 3.3 times as likely to die of heart disease. Glucose levels in the 70 to 79 range increased risk by 2.4 times. The heart-healthy range was between 80 and 109. As levels went over 109, risk began to increase.

This was no small study. It was very well designed and involved more than 40,000 patients. Take a close look at your laboratory report. Don't take your doctor's word for it that you're "just fine." You have a right to examine your own records, and you definitely should. It's one more example of playing an active role in protecting your own health.

Don't be too disturbed if your physician is unaware of the CHD risks of high uric acid and low glucose levels. This is new information and few doctors outside of cardiology read all the heart journals. If you'd like to tell your doctor about them, I've cited both studies in the references for this chapter.

DIABETES AND HEART DISEASE

In addition to other, more publicized risk factors, diabetes places its sufferers at a particularly high risk of heart disease. That additional risk is much higher for women than men. In fact, just having diabetes totally wipes out the protection against CHD most women enjoy until menopause, putting them at as much risk as men or more.

There are two types of diabetes. Type 1, which was previously termed juvenile diabetes, typically occurs earlier in life and involves an inability of the pancreas to make enough insulin to spark glucose into the body's cells for energy. Type 1 diabetics generally must have daily injections of insulin. Type 2 diabetes, earlier called mature-onset diabetes, strikes later in life, although a frightening increase in the disease has occurred in teenagers and people in their twenties. In this form of diabetes, the pancreas produces insulin but the body becomes resistant to it. In both types, glucose builds up in the blood. The diagnosis of diabetes is made when blood sugar levels go above 126.

More than 85 percent of men and women who develop type 2 diabetes are overweight and sedentary. As these two problems have become more common in our society, incidence of diabetes has increased. And with that rise comes a jump in CHD risk.

The Rancho Bernardo study, an ongoing project of the University of California at San Diego, has provided some deadly specifics. A total of 207 men and 1276 women with Type 2 diabetes were compared with 2137 adults without the disease. Women with diabetes had 3.3 times the risk of heart disease as those without the disease. Diabetes increased CHD risk in men 1.8 times.

In a very real way, Type 2 diabetes is a wonderful disease to have. That's because the vast majority of men and women who develop Type 2 diabetes can make it go away. You sure can't say that about most diseases!

The secret to banishing Type 2 diabetes is very simple, yet few diabetic men and women take advantage of it. The ultimate prescription consists of increased physical activity and weight loss. Time and time again, doctors have proven that when a patient loses weight and does regular exercise, glucose levels fall below 126, ideally down to about 100 or so. Hard to do? Sure it is. Giving up one's old habits and replacing them with healthy ones takes commitment.

But, wow, that investment in health pays off great dividends. In addition to the increased risk of heart disease, diabetes brings with it the threat of blindness, kidney failure, impotence for men, and possible amputation of the feet owing to gangrene brought on by impaired circulation. Get rid of diabetes and you get rid of all those problems.

Is that gooey dessert really worth the loss of sight? Wouldn't you be willing to take a long walk daily to prevent heart disease? There's an old saying: "I'd give an arm and a leg" for this or that. Would you give a foot, or both feet, just to stay overweight and inactive?

Now back to some specifics.

Cholesterol levels are particularly important for diabetic patients. Type 2 diabetics are at special risk when levels of the protective HDL are low and triglycerides and LDL are high. The risk of death, as published in the American Heart Association's official journal, is four times as great for such individuals.

Type 2 diabetes patients have elevated levels of glucose in the blood since their insulin is unable to facilitate the cells' use of blood glucose. As a result, their bodies produce additional insulin to compensate, leading to the condition known as hyperinsulinemia, which means too much insulin in the blood. But such individuals are insulin-resistant, and even excessive levels do not decrease sugar loads. Now doctors are recognizing that those excessive insulin levels are themselves at least partially responsible for the diabetic patient's increased CHD risk.

Insulin resistance has gotten a lot of press in books, magazines, and newspapers. But it is extremely important to note that insulin resistance *does not* lead to obesity. It's the other way around. As one remains overweight and sedentary over a period of time (no, it doesn't happen right away), the body becomes more and more insulin-resistant. Eventually that resistance leads to a buildup of glucose in the blood and the development of diabetes and its attendant risks.

Insulin resistance is accompanied by a constellation of risks, including elevated triglycerides, lowered HDL counts, and high blood pressure. Previously, doctors thought it was those accompanying factors that were responsible for added risk. Now the higher-than-normal levels of insulin in the blood themselves are seen as dangerous.

Testing for insulin resistance is not commonly performed, as it is both expensive and time-consuming. To do so, doctors administer glucose and insulin intravenously over at least three hours to determine how much insulin is required to maintain a constant normal level of blood sugar. This is called the glucose clamp technique.

Results are fed into a computer programmed to calculate the body's response to the insulin.

Further aggravating the problem, some medications used to treat high blood pressure and correct cholesterol and other lipid elevations actually result in raising insulin levels. And in some cases, when diabetic patients are unable to control glucose levels by way of diet, exercise, and oral medications, doctors may prescribe insulin injections to lower sugar counts. That extra insulin may in itself lead to increased risk of heart disease. And once one begins to take insulin injections, it's extremely difficult to get rid of them. It becomes a vicious circle, but one you can avoid with simple lifestyle modifications.

Approximately 16 million Americans have diabetes. It is often said that half of all diabetics remain undiagnosed. Diabetes is the fourth leading cause of death in the United States. Because of damage done by diabetes to nerve endings, patients may not sense the symptoms of heart disease such as angina or chest pain and the disease goes untreated or worsens. Moreover, diabetic patients suffer from impaired function of the left ventricle of the heart, the pumping chamber. Such individuals benefit from drugs such as aspirin, beta blockers, and ACE inhibitors even more than those without diabetes.

Diabetes kills. Don't be a victim. Fight for your life by making that commitment to weight loss and regular exercise today, right now. You'll find all the information you need in this book.

THYROID PROBLEMS

The thyroid gland, located in the throat, plays a very important role in maintaining health and function throughout our lives. This relatively small gland produces a hormone that influences every cell, tissue, and organ in the body. The thyroid regulates the body's metabolism and affects heart rate, energy, and mood. Its impact on heart disease has become more clearly understood during the past few years.

In a huge study to determine the incidence of thyroid problems, doctors learned that there may be more than 13 million Americans who are unaware that they have a thyroid condition. That's double the number previously believed. Researchers also determined that even the slightest decrease in thyroid function may increase cholesterol levels, thus increasing risk of heart disease. Here's the sad fact: even someone doing his or her best to eat the right foods may have a high cholesterol level because of an underactive thyroid of which he or she is totally unaware.

Impaired thyroid function, known as hypothyroidism, may or may not have clear signs and symptoms, at least during the early stages of decline. But as the thyroid produces less hormone, cholesterol levels rise. Average levels found in persons with full-blown hypothyroidism were 251, while those with far lesser thyroid inactivity were 224—more than enough to put someone at significant risk.

Symptoms include fatigue, depression, forgetfulness, unexplained weight gain, and menstrual irregularities. But those warning signs are shared by many other disorders, and by simple aging. For women, untreated hypothyroidism may lead not only to heart disease but also to osteoporosis and infertility.

While thyroid problems can occur at any time in a person's life, incidence increases with age. One woman in eight will develop a thyroid disorder during her lifetime. By age 60, more than 20 percent of all American women will have a thyroid disturbance.

Testing and treatment are both very simple. Many doctors now believe that those with high cholesterol levels should be tested by measuring the amount of thyroid hormone in the blood. If the thyroid gland is inactive, a daily dose of additional thyroid hormone can be taken with no unpleasant side effects or adverse reactions. In fact, those who start taking the tiny little pills feel much better in short order. They sleep better, have more energy, are less irritable, and may even lose some unwanted pounds and inches. And the long-term benefits of CHD prevention are enormous.

IRONCLAD ARTERIES?

Got "iron-poor" blood? An increasing number of heart researchers think that's a good thing. For the past few years the idea that too much iron in the blood might be linked with heart disease became quite controversial. One study noted a correlation while another found no connection. The research and opinions went back and forth. Now the balance seems to tilt in a specific direction, and you and I might want to pay attention to the iron levels in our bloodstream.

A doctor in Florida began the controversy in 1981, but very few heard about his theory until the mid-1990s. Dr. Jerome Sullivan, at the University of Florida, hypothesized that women might be protected against heart disease in part because of their loss of iron through menstruation. Postmenopausal women no longer removing iron from the blood on a monthly basis began to increase their CHD risk. Men, on the other hand, begin to increase the level of iron in their blood by about age 20, and it is at that age that heart disease risk begins to increase for them. Or so the thinking went.

Researchers in Finland jumped into the fray with studies showing a definite link. American investigations were not nearly as clear in indicting the mineral. I myself questioned the iron theory in my quarterly newsletter over the years. For one thing, I was skeptical about the leading Finnish researcher's enthusiasm since he himself has the condition known as hemochromatosis, in which unnaturally high levels of iron build up in the blood. As recently as February 1999, a major review of studies on iron and heart disease failed to demonstrate a clear-cut association between iron status and CHD.

The flip side of the argument shows a somewhat stronger link. A study presented in October 2000 at a heart conference showed that iron can damage the endothelium, the lining of the arteries. Such damage lessens the arteries' ability to dilate to allow for greater blood flow when needed. Healthy volunteers were injected with high doses of iron, and ultrasound was used to examine the function of the endothelium. Indeed, arteries were impaired in their dilation capabilities.

The same researchers then wondered whether reducing iron levels could improve endothelial function. They gave volunteers a chemical that depletes stored iron. Afterward, endothelial dilation got better. The investigators speculate that iron does its damage by interfering with the action of nitric oxide (NO), a chemical released by the endothelium. This causes the blood vessels to relax in order to accommodate increased blood flow required during physical or emotional stress. Iron also increases levels of another chemical that causes oxidation.

Is the iron debate settled? I'm sure that many more papers will get published in the coming years on both sides of the dispute. But in this case, it's extremely easy to play it safe.

First, no male past the age of 20 needs any more iron than is supplied by the average American diet, even by a diet that cuts back on red meat, which is the principal source of the mineral. The 16 mg typically found in daily vitamin-mineral supplements probably would do no real harm, but then again, it would do no good, either. Fortunately, some supplements come in iron-free formulations. That's what I take.

One in about 250 people have a genetic condition that leads to hemochromatosis. Such individuals have double the normal ability to absorb iron from the diet, and the iron builds up in the blood. Hemochromatosis patients have symptoms including fatigue and unexplained weight gain, and have a much higher risk of dying of heart disease or stroke. Treatment for hemochromatosis consists of regular bloodletting; unfortunately, the blood cannot be used for transfusions and is discarded.

But anyone can potentially reduce the risk posed by stored iron by donating blood. Regardless of the amount of iron stored in the blood, such regular donations will bring the mineral down to safe levels while doing something nice for society. Studies have hinted that those who contribute blood have less CHD risk.

As for women of childbearing age, nature takes care of any iron surplus. If anything, premenopausal women tend to be deficient and should take daily supplements. After menopause, contributing blood would be wise, just to stay on the safe side. My wife does so at least twice a year, and she no longer takes iron supplements.

IT'S OK TO BE PHOBIC ABOUT HOMOCYSTEINE

Back in 1984, following that second bypass surgery, I started taking my health really seriously. In addition to the regimen that lowered my cholesterol level, I began a complete program of dietary supplements. One of the tablets I swallowed each morning was a vitamin B complex formulation. Without even thinking about it, that simple decision was one of the things that saved my life.

It turns out that three B vitamins—folic acid, B_6, and B_{12}—are essential in the metabolic breakdown of proteins into amino acids. Without enough of those B vitamins, one particular amino acid, homocysteine, is not properly metabolized and builds up in the blood. High levels of homocysteine have now been solidly linked with increased risk of CHD. This is known as an independent risk factor; that is to say, elevated homocysteine leads to heart disease even in the absence of other factors such as diabetes, smoking, or hypertension.

The story began more than 30 years ago, although the research done by Dr. Kilmer McCulley remained obscure for decades. At that time he noticed that an infant with a genetic metabolic problem that led to a rise in homocysteine in the blood had severe atherosclerosis when an autopsy was done after the child's death. Later investigations found that in patients with hyperhomocysteinemia—a rare genetic condition that results in elevated amounts of homocysteine in the blood—usually died of premature heart attacks.

But because these were rare instances, they didn't get much

attention in cardiology circles. Then researchers around the world began measuring levels of homocysteine in men and women and correlating those counts with incidence of fatal and nonfatal heart attacks. Most of the studies showed a distinct connection.

Men more frequently exhibit elevated homocysteine levels, but the condition afflicts both sexes. Certainly there is a genetic component that determines just how efficiently one breaks down the amino acid, but the principal problem appears to be dietary insufficiencies, if not deficiencies, of the three B vitamins, particularly folic acid. And as we age, homocysteine levels tend to climb. Nearly one-third of all patients followed in the long-term Framingham Heart Study who were over the age of 67 had a high level of the substance in the blood.

The landmark study of homocysteine came out of the data collected from 271 male physicians participating in a huge prospective study. A prospective study is one in which subjects are healthy at the beginning of the observation, but as bad things happened to them, scientists tried to figure out what they have in common. In this case, men whose homocysteine levels were in the highest 5 percent were more than three times at risk of having a heart attack, even after eliminating all other risk factors. Pooling the data from all recent investigations indicates that homocysteine concentrations are about 30 percent higher than normal in people who develop heart disease.

There have been dozens, if not hundreds, of studies showing a clear association between elevated homocysteine levels and both heart attack and stroke. Here are just a few of the results of those studies:

- Women in the Nurses' Health Study with high counts of homocysteine had twice the risk of all cardiovascular events, including heart attack, stroke, bypass surgery, and angioplasty, compared with those with lower levels. Previous data from that study showed that nurses who consumed the most folic acid and B_6 slashed their CHD risk.
- Children whose parents were diagnosed with CHD are likely to have increased homocysteine levels, regardless of sex or race.
- In patients who had angiograms that revealed clogged arteries, homocysteine levels correlated directly with fatal heart attacks.
- Homocysteine multiplies the danger of established risk factors such as smoking, hypertension, and high cholesterol.
- Combating high homocysteine levels with B vitamin supplementation halted the rate of progression of atherosclerosis. Another study showed that subjects whose previously high

levels of homocysteine were lowered brought their CHD risk down to that of those who had normal counts to begin with.

■ As with cholesterol, the higher the homocysteine level, the greater the risk.

High levels of homocysteine lead to trouble in a number of ways. Damage to the endothelial lining of the arteries leads to the formation of plaque. The amino acid stimulates excessive growth of smooth muscle cells, causing the plaque to grow. And homocysteine is frequently responsible for the rupture of plaque and the subsequent formation of blood clots, which precipitate heart attacks. Homocysteine also results in accelerated production of collagen, a major component of atherosclerotic plaque, which, in turn, causes the plaque to increase in size.

Most doctors don't routinely test their patients for homocysteine levels, although that may change in the coming years. At this point, many insurance companies are reluctant to pay for the test. But the real question is whether testing is actually necessary. More about the logic behind that shortly.

Normal levels for homocysteine are from 9 to 10 micromoles per liter (μmol/L). As with cholesterol, risk gradually increases as the number goes up. At levels of 14 to 15 and more, homocysteine represents an independent risk factor and magnifies the effect of other risk factors.

The good news about this new villain in the CHD picture is that homocysteine can easily be controlled by consuming adequate amounts of the three B vitamins. Until very recently the question has been not whether this is effective, since it has been clinically documented any number of times, but rather, how much is enough.

The level of folic acid recommended by U.S. federal authorities was reduced from 400 micrograms (μg) daily to 200 μg a number of years ago. Some believe that the reduction in folic acid intake has been partially responsible for both heart attacks and a birth defect known as spina bifida. The recommendation was brought back to 400 μg in the late 1990s.

Meanwhile, scientists were trying to determine how much folic acid would be needed to normalize homocysteine. For some individuals, 400 μg was not enough, so doctors gave them ten times that amount or more. The most recent research, presented at the 2000 meeting of the American Heart Association, demonstrates that a maximal dosage of 800 μg is sufficient for the vast majority of patients, and definitely not more than 1200 μg.

To put that into perspective, the typical vitamin-mineral supplement contains 400 µg. B complex supplements contain that amount or more. So if one were to take a daily vitamin-mineral tablet in the morning with breakfast and a B complex tablet sometime later in the day, that would provide adequate folic acid to bring homocysteine into the healthy zone.

Moreover, such supplementation would ensure you get vitamins B_6 and B_{12} as well. The recommended daily intake of B_6 is 2 mg and that of B_{12} is 6 µg. The three vitmains—folic acid, B_6, and B_{12}—appear to work best together as a defense against homocysteine. In fact, some research has shown that inadequate intake of B_6 may in itself compromise heart health. Moreover, some individuals, especially vegetarians but also those severely restricting consumption of red meat, may be deficient in B_{12}. There's no need to pay extra money for supplements specifically labeled as "specially formulated" to protect against homocysteine and CHD risk. Any supplements providing folic acid, B_6, and B_{12} will do very nicely.

Currently, the American Heart Association does not recommend supplements, preferring instead to advise daily consumption of foods that provide those nutrients. And, yes, it is possible to achieve at least minimum levels of intake by diet alone. But it may not be easy and it may not be enough.

By all means, start with the diet. Make sure that you eat lots of fruits and vegetables, which are excellent sources of folate (the form of the B vitamin found in food, as compared with folic acid, which is found in supplements and fortified foods). The same goes for beans and lentils of all sorts. And beginning in 1998, federal authorities mandated that flour, breads, and cereals be fortified with folic acid. But that amount still leaves homocysteine levels higher than desirable for many individuals.

View tablets for what they are: supplements, not alternatives, to food. Supplementing a good diet with a daily vitamin-mineral tablet and a B complex tablet will provide enough folic acid, B_6, and B_{12} to completely eliminate homocysteine as a risk factor.

Which brings us back to testing. Let's say that a homocysteine test reveals your count at, say, 13 or 14. What will you do? Take the B vitamin trio, of course. If you were to have another test in a couple of months, you'd find that your homocysteine measurement would come down to the safe 9 to 10 zone. And you'd keep taking the supplements for the rest of your life.

So why bother with the testing in the first place? Supplementation with B vitamins at the levels I've been discussing can do no harm and are likely to do a lot of good by protecting against high homocysteine levels, keeping women from giving birth to babies with spina bifida, and promoting general good health. Of course, the ultimate decision to test or not to test should be made after a discussion with your own doctor.

BLOOD CLOTS AND HEART DISEASE

Our bodies continuously form and dissolve clots in our bloodstreams. It's a natural, normal process. In fact, if you and I lacked the ability to clot, we'd bleed to death from the slightest cuts. But clots also have a dark side, precipitating heart attacks and strokes.

A number of factors come into play in the body's balancing act of forming and dissolving clots. As the specialized blood cells known as platelets gather together (platelet aggregation), they tend to form clots. The more they aggregate, the more and bigger clots. There's a whole physiological menu of substances involved in the clotting process. When I took my graduate training in physiology, we had to memorize each of those clotting factors, but I won't confuse you with all their names and functions. Suffice it to say that a major player is a substance called fibrinogen, which is absolutely essential for getting clots started.

On the other side of the equation, the body has a number of ways to break down clots as needed. You may have heard of the clot-busting drug tPA, which is injected into the arteries of patients suffering a heart attack to return normal blood flow to the heart. The body produces its own supply of tissue plasminogen activator (tPA) to keep clots under control. And, just as there are a number of factors involved with forming clots, there are substances in the blood designed to break them down. That process is called fibrinolysis.

Everything's fine as long as the equation stays balanced. Clots form, clots dissolve. But too much of one substance or too little of another, and the balance gets thrown out of whack and excessive clot formation occurs. Needless to say, that's a bad thing, because it accelerates the progression of atherosclerosis and increases the risk of heart attack and stroke.

Elevated fibrinogen levels have been established as an independent risk factor for CHD from large, long-term studies in both the United States and Britain. Conversely, low levels of fibrinogen appear to protect against CHD. A number of factors determine fibrinogen levels, including age, smoking, physical activity, obesity, diabetes, excessive insulin, and lipids—both LDL and triglycerides. Light to moderate alcohol intake appears to reduce fibrinogen levels.

So what do you do about all this? Definitely quit smoking, lose weight if necessary, increase physical activity, reduce lipid levels, and take steps to control diabetes and insulin levels. If you enjoy a drink or two a day, fine, but this isn't a reason to start drinking. And don't forget that more than moderate drinking damages the heart rather than protecting it.

As you know already, I'm a big fan of the vitamin niacin. I've devoted a whole chapter to it. That's because it does so much more than just lower LDL cholesterol. And one of the things it does is reduce fibrinogen levels. Yes, niacin can protect you, as it does me, from developing potentially fatal blood clots. Pretty important.

And what about platelet aggregation? Needless to say, it would be nice to prevent excessive gathering of platelets and clot formation. Happily, there are a number of ways to do just that.

Those who regularly eat fish, especially fatty fish, have special CHD protection. That's because the omega-3 fatty acids in fish lessen clotting, largely by reducing platelet aggregation. In fact, Inuit peoples, who consume huge amounts of those omega-3 fats, tend to bruise very easily.

Research published in 2000 revealed that alcohol's protective benefits include reduction of platelet aggregation. Again, the watchword is moderation.

Next, we have aspirin. We've all heard how a daily aspirin tablet protects against heart attacks. It does so both by reducing platelet aggregation and by promoting fibrinolysis—the breakdown of clots. While there is still some controversy about the ideal dosage, the American Heart Association recommends a baby aspirin containing 81 mg of aspirin daily, with a twice-monthly booster of a standard 350-mg tablet. Others believe that the 350-mg tablet daily is the better bet for those who can tolerate it without gastric upset. I've been taking that amount every single day since my second bypass in 1984.*

INFLAMMATION AND CHD

For many years, doctors have hypothesized that the atherosclerotic process of clogging the arteries begins with a response of the endothe-

---

*Only aspirin has this protective effect, not any of the anti-inflammatory aspirin alternatives such as Tylenol, Advil, or Naprosyn.

lial lining of those arteries to an injury of some sort. Picture the inside of the artery getting nicked or damaged. The body then tries to patch up that injury with a concretion of cholesterol, smooth muscle cells, and specialized white blood cells. With a sufficient amount of cholesterol floating around in the bloodstream, the plaque formed in this way continues to grow and grow.

We've been going over some of the ways we can protect the endothelial lining and prevent the buildup of plaque. Obviously, without sufficient building materials such as Lp(a) and LDL cholesterol, especially in its oxidized form, plaque won't develop as readily. And we have lots of evidence that by reducing levels of those lipids we can, in fact, virtually halt the progression of the disease.

In the years to come, we can hope that doctors will figure out just what causes endothelial injuries and the resultant inflammation, which, in turn, leads to atherosclerosis. In the meantime, however, research has at least given us a way to determine whether such inflammation is present in the arteries. That's done by measuring levels of a substance called C-reactive protein (CRP).

In the past few years, studies done all over the world have indicated that CRP is a powerful predictor of CHD and the risk of heart attack and stroke in both men and women. The abbreviated hs-CRP test, which has a high sensitivity to levels of CRP different from those typical in other inflammatory processes such as arthritis, is readily available through any doctor's office at a reasonably low price. Many authorities believe that hs-CRP should become as routine as cholesterol testing and is even better at zeroing in on those men and women who are at particularly high risk.

Research has shown a linear progression between increased levels of CRP and atherosclerotic blockage and risk of heart attck and/or stroke. Compare your own test results with the following breakdown:

less than 0.70 mg/dL	lowest risk
0.70 to 1.1 mg/dL	low risk
1.2 to 1.9 mg/dL	average risk
2.0 to 3.8 mg/dL	higher risk
3.9 to 15.0 mg/dL	highest risk

The big question on the minds of cardiologists is what to do about elevated CRP. A few believe that it would be a good thing to bring CRP levels down, perhaps by anti-inflammatory agents, including aspirin. Maybe that is one way that aspirin does, in fact, protect against CHD and heart attacks. Preliminary data hint that statin cholesterol-lowering drugs reduce CRP counts. But is that a result of cholesterol reduction or of some currently unknown action of the statins? Probably the former, but time will tell.

The majority of doctors feel that CRP elevations should flash a warning signal to alert both patient and physician to the increased importance of controlling the risk factors that we absolutely know contribute to atherosclerotic development and progression and to risk of fatal and nonfatal MIs and strokes. That means aggressive cholesterol lowering, hypertension control, cigarette cessation, diabetes control, and dealing with all the other controllable things we've been going over in this chapter.

There is no current evidence that CRP plays an active role in the development and progression of CHD. Rather, it acts as what is called a "marker" for disease. Compare it to a red warning light that appears on the instrumental panel of your car. You don't try to figure out how to make that red light go away. You fix the underlying problem.

GETTING THE BUGS OUT:
THE GERM THEORY OF HEART DISEASE

It may be that the inflammation detected by the hs-CRP test may be caused, at least in part, by infection with some sort of bacteria or virus. Indeed, perhaps some bug is ultimately responsible for heart disease itself. Does this sound way-out? Let's consider the history of germ theory.

Louis Pasteur showed us how bacteria causes milk to go bad, and today pasteurized milk is the norm. In 1867 the English surgeon Joseph Lister proved that antiseptic procedures made "clean" surgery less lethal for patients. Ignaz Semmelweis did the same for childbirth, saving mothers' lives by chiding physicians to wash their hands.

Far more recently, the Australian physician Barry Marshall demonstrated that ulcers were caused not by stress or spicy foods but rather by a common bacterium called *Helicobacter pylori*. When doctors ignored his initial research findings, Dr. Marshall drank solutions of *H. pylori* and gave himself ulcers, which he then cured with antibiotics. Coincidentally, I was at the scientific conference where he introduced his ideas in the mid-1980s.

For that reason, I've been particularly attentive to research articles in the medical literature addressing potential links between CHD and one germ or another. Might the injury that causes the inflammation that leads to plaque formation be caused by a microbe?

The germ theory of heart disease presents a good example of the scientific process. Remember the old Indian tale of the three blind men who encounter an elephant? One touches the animal's side and says the beast must be like a wall; the second man, grasping the trunk, proclaims the elephant to be a large snake; and the third man, putting his arms around the leg, believes the creature to be like a tree.

The scientific process consists of taking pieces here and there and putting them together to form a mosaic. No one piece represents the whole, nor can it hint at what the mosaic portrays.

So here we are with the idea that a number of microbes, including *H. pylori* (the one that causes ulcers), *Chlamydia pneumoniae* (bacteria responsible for various diseases), *Herpes simplex* (the virus behind cold sores), cytomegalovirus (CMV, a bug involved in an infection that resembles mononucleosis, the so-called kissing disease), and the bacteria resulting in periodontal disease in the gum tissue surrounding the teeth, might have something to do with the formation and development of atherosclerosis. As with the blind men, various scientists have published data in the world's most prestigious medical journals indicting or vindicating each of those bacteria and viruses.

On the positive side, doctors at the Cardiovascular Research Institute in Washington, D.C., concluded that cytomegalovirus is an independent risk factor for CHD in women. A paper published by Italian researchers that linked particularly nasty strains of *H. pylori* with CHD was accompanied by an editorial praising the quality of the investigation techniques and the promise of its conclusions. After looking at samples of the tissue removed from diseased arteries, another research group found *C. pneumoniae* in 73 percent, compared with only 4 percent of samples taken from normal, healthy arteries. And a paper presented at the 2000 AHA meeting concluded that gum disease may predict heart disease since, in the patients examined, 85 percent of those entering the hospital with a heart attack had periodontal disease, compared with 29 percent of individuals free of disease.

The one thing all these papers and editorials have in common is a call for physicians not to rush to give their patients antibiotics. More about such treatment shortly. But first, let's look at some of the negative conclusions in other studies.

Two large investigations, involving 21,520 and 5661 men respectively, found that *C. pneumoniae* was no more prevalent in those with CHD than those without heart disease. Similarly, German doctors failed to show a correlation between *H. pylori* and CHD after other risk factors were taken into statistical consideration. Another German study did find *C. pneumoniae*, but not CMV, in occluded bypass

vein grafts. Finally, a study concluded adamantly that periodontal disease was not linked with CHD in the patients examined.

So why bother you with such details? Because when you see a
newspaper report saying yes to the germ theory of CHD, remember
that the next study just very well might say no. Unfortunately, newspapers and magazines are notorious for writing about those positive,
gee-whiz findings and ignoring the negative ones. Sadly, researchers
confide, it's the same with scientific journals!

At this point no doctor should prescribe antibiotics to treat bacteria
or viruses. Nor should they bother to test you for their presence. We
don't know as yet which microbe, if any, is the responsible culprit, nor
do we know how much antibiotic should be given, or for how long.

Large-scale studies involving several thousands of heart disease
patients are now under way, and preliminary data will start coming in
in about two years.

Personally, I'm keeping my fingers crossed that the ongoing investigations do come up with a microbial cause of heart disease.
Wouldn't it be terrific if a vaccine could be developed that would protect the public, especially those with a family history of CHD?

SOME WEIRD RISK FACTORS

Perhaps you read in the papers that bald men are at greater risk for
heart disease than those with a full head of hair. Another study
pointed the finger of fate at short men, who were said to be in more
danger than those of greater stature. Recently, women with a snoring
problem were reported to have a greater risk for getting heart disease.
Dazed and confused? It's time to put these things, and some others,
into proper perspective.

Ultimately, it comes down to defining a couple of terms. First, the
term "marker." This is used to designate a factor that has been *associated* with a disease. Changing such a marker, however, would have no
effect on risk. Giving a bald man a hair transplant, for example,
would not alter his cardiovascular risk. Baldness is simply a marker
for underlying and associated conditions; in this case, probably tes-
tosterone levels come into play.

We learned about CRP a few pages ago. Right now, it's considered
a potent predictor of heart disease, a marker, for some underlying
situation, maybe bacteria, maybe something else. If, as time goes on,
we find out that by treating and reducing the inflammation signaled
by CRP we can reduce the development of atherosclerosis and the
occurrence of heart attacks, it will become a risk factor.

What about those snoring women? As reported in the February 2000 issue of the *Journal of the American College of Cardiology,* women who snore regularly have about twice the risk of heart attacks and strokes of those who sleep silently. That association comes from studying nearly 72,000 female nurses aged 40 to 65 at the beginning of the investigation. Would treating their snoring eliminate the cardiovascular risk? Probably not, unless the snoring was the result of apnea, in wihch one periodically stops breathing. The snoring is likely a marker for an underlying condition—in this case, probably excess weight that results in snoring but that also influences heart disease.

The list of such markers is quite long, including some things that doctors haven't quite figured out, such as creases in the lobes of one's ears, statistically associated with greater odds of developing heart disease. My friend, Dr. Jack Sternlieb, says that the vast majority of patients on whom he has performed bypass surgery have had those ear creases.

All those markers just give doctors and their patients a signal that such individuals should pay more attention to things that *can* influence the development of heart disease. That, in turn, brings us to defining a risk factor in heart disease. Such factors include cholesterol levels, blood pressure, diabetes, obesity, sedentary behavior, and so forth. Most of these factors—we can't do much about our ages or gender—can be altered, and doing so can and will reduce risk. And while we can't turn back our chronological age, we certainly can affect our physiological age by increasing levels of physical activity, quitting smoking, and eating better.

So for those of you who happen to be bald, short, ear-creased snorers, let those markers motivate you to get more exercise, lose any extra pounds, and keep that cholesterol under control. And don't forget that it's all a matter of statistics. At age 35, I was slender, had a full head of hair (I still do), never snored, and had ear lobes without creases. But I had a heart attack that year, along with bypass surgery. Six years later I had my second bypass and finally got religion regarding the risk factors that really *do* matter.

2
Special Considerations for Women, the Young, and the Elderly

Early research in heart disease focused almost entirely on middle-aged men. Until the late 1980s and early 1990s, anyone else had to assume recommendations for men would benefit them as well. Fortunately, times have changed, and now it's appropriate to consider the special needs of women, children and young adults, and the elderly.

WOMEN AND HEART DISEASE

Even today the average woman fears cancer far more than heart disease. Yet while one in eight women will develop breast cancer, and far fewer are afflicted with ovarian and uterine cancer, one in two will develop heart disease. Half of all American women, and half of all women in westernized countries, die of heart disease.

Yes, a lot more attention has been paid to this deadly fact in the media, research in recent years has focused on women and heart disease, and doctors are more aware of the problem. But the right information has not trickled down to women themselves. As a result, heart disease remains the number one killer of women.

For openers, the disease is not diagnosed as early in women as it is in men; neither women nor their doctors pay a lot of attention to it. When heart attacks do occur, they are more serious and more often fatal than in men. Women who do survive frequently suffer damaged hearts, and quality of life declines more than for men. Angioplasty and bypass surgery rates are far lower for women.

So much for the grim statistics. What can women do to protect themselves from this killer? A lot!

Start with testing. Are you aware of your current risk factors, including total cholesterol, LDL and HDL levels, triglycerides, blood pressure, glucose levels? Especially if you have a family history of CHD, have you been evaluated by such tests as the treadmill exercise test, ultrafast CT to detect calcium in the arteries, perhaps even more sophisticated exams including echocardiogram and angiography?

Women have had to fight for everything men take for granted, such as equal pay for equal work. Sadly, you have to fight to protect your health and your life as well. That means going to your doctor and demanding a complete and thorough heart-health workup.

For most women, menopause marks the time when they start to catch up with men in the development of atherosclerosis. A number of factors come into play, including elevations in total and LDL cholesterol and the superdeadly LDL variant known as Lp(a), and decreases in the protective HDL.

Unfortunately, the use of the female hormone, estrogen, while preventing CHD, increases the risk of breast and endometrial cancers. But the good news is that combining estrogen with progestin blocks the ill effects while still providing the benefits.

Moreover, doctors now have a drug called raloxifene, which decreases LDL cholesterol, Lp(a), and the occurrence of blood clots. Raloxifene also offers protection against the bone demineralizing disease osteoporosis, as does HRT. But the new drug is not as effective in raising HDL or lowering the Lp(a). To complement raloxifene, therefore, you might want to add niacin to your regimen, which will most effectively raise HDL, lower Lp(a) and triglycerides, and provide even more lowering of LDL cholesterol. Again, discuss this with your doctor.

Many women, having heard of the potential downside of HRT, turn to various "natural" remedies found in health food stores. Be aware, however, that some, such as those derived from yams, have an estrogen-promoting effect that can be equal to that of HRT itself.

It appears that one reason women are protected from heart disease until menopause has to do with lower levels of an enzyme called hepatic lipase, which breaks down a component in the body's cholesterol manufacture. The more hepatic lipase the body produces, the more LDL cholesterol it can turn out in the liver, and in the particularly dangerous small, dense particle form. Men, unhappily, have a lot more hepatic lipase than women—that is, until women hit menopause, when their bodies start churning out the enzyme.

Until 2001, women and their doctors placed tremendous faith in the ability of hormone therapy (HRT) to protect against heart disease after menopause. Estrogen raised levels of the protective HDL cholesterol while reducing artery-clogging LDL and Lp(a). Observational studies showed that women receiving HRT had less heart disease and fewer deaths from heart attacks than those who did not take the hormones.

But then a study showed that for women with pre-existing CHD, HRT did not reduce subsequent heart attacks or strokes. Doctors held out hope that HRT might prevent heart disease when initiated prior to the development of CHD.

The second shoe dropped in the summer of 2002. The Women's Health Initiative (WHI) was an 8-year study, part of which looked at the role of HRT in the health of post-menopausal women. Participants got either HRT or placebos. Those women did not have diagnosed CHD at the beginning of the study. Hopes were high that HRT would be definitively established as being protective.

But that segment of the WHI was prematurely halted after just five years when it appeared that rather than lessening risk, HRT actually increased the incidence of heart attack and stroke, albeit just slightly.

Doctors now suggest HRT only for short periods of time, in small dosages, to reduce symptoms at the onset of menopause. Protection against heart disease should come from regular exercise, a healthy diet, and reduction of established risk factors including elevated blood pressure, cholesterol, homocysteine, and others. Sorry, HRT is not the magic pill we had hoped for.

AN OUNCE OF PREVENTION

Ideally, women should start taking preventive measures against CHD way before menopause. However, it's never too late to make life-saving behavior modifications. The power of prevention was dramatically presented in the *New England Journal of Medicine* in August 2000.

Doctors had been tracking the health of women enrolled in the Nurses' Health Study for 14 years. During those years, the researchers compared the nurses' lifestyle patterns with the incidence of coronary events, including heart attacks and death. Average risk was assigned the number 1.0. Women at greater than average risk were over 1.0, those with less risk had a lower risk-ratio number; for example, women at twice the risk of having a coronary event would be listed at 2.0. Well, there was one group of women whose risk-ratio was a mere 0.17!

Who were those lucky ladies? They most closely complied with the five healthy lifestyle parameters the doctors kept track of. They were nonsmokers. They drank alcohol moderately. They maintained healthy body weight. They exercised at least half an hour daily. And they ate healthy diets that included plenty of fiber, fish, fresh fruits and vegetables, and far more poly- and monounsaturated than saturated fats.

Women in the study were 34 to 59 years old at the start. During the 14 years, the percentage of smokers dropped by 41 percent. Those are good signs of what women in general are doing. Unfortunately, the number of women who were considered overweight or obese increased by 39 percent, although the dietary profile of foods consumed improved in terms of fat, fiber, and so forth.

Over the span of those 14 years, the incidence of coronary events dropped by 21 percent. On the other hand, the increase in the number of overweight and obese women accounted for an 8 percent *increase* in CHD.

The study did not take into consideration other potentially beneficial behaviors such as antioxidant intake other than through food or the use of B vitamins to combat the risk factor of homocysteine. Interestingly, the researchers believe that women can actually reduce their risk ratio to even less than 0.17 by closer long-term compliance with heart-healthy lifestyle behaviors. And, of course, it's never too late to start making improvements. You bought this book and you are reading this chapter. Now put the recommendations into effect, starting today, if you haven't already done so.

Get your cholesterol level down well below 200, ideally in the 160 to 180 range with an LDL of 100 or lower. Walk or do other physical activity regularly. Control your blood pressure and, if you have it, diabetes. Maintain a healthy body weight. Definitely quit smoking and avoid passive smoke intake.

CHILDREN, TEENS, AND YOUNG ADULTS

Heart disease had long been viewed as a problem for middle-aged and older men. Certainly we know now that women must also protect themselves against CHD. And today, doctors recognize that heart disease begins in childhood.

My own experience began with my son and daughter, who were 9 and 6 years old, respectively, when my book came out in 1987. Becoming more and more involved with ongoing research and developments, I was soon aware that Ross and Jenny should have their cholesterol levels checked. Indeed, Ross's was elevated for his age.

From that point forward, a heart-healthy lifestyle became a way of life for the entire family, not just for me. We shopped for food together, getting them involved from point of purchase to the kitchen to restaurants to parties. I also urged physical activity and encouraged sports and exercise almost as much as schoolwork.

Then came the teen years, with all the usual complications. And today, Ross and Jenny are entering young adulthood. Of course I've tracked the research on CHD and the young throughout the years. I'm happy to say that both my children's risk factors for CHD, including cholesterol but far beyond, are totally under control. With that in mind, let's take a look at the need for preventive measures at each stage of life.

Heart Disease Begins in Childhood

That's the statement I first heard from Dr. Gerald Berenson, who heads up the famed Bogalusa, Louisiana, children's heart study. Having tracked a large number of black and white boys and girls for many years, carefully measuring growth, blood pressure, cholesterol, and smoking and exercise habits, Dr. Berenson and his coworkers found that kids as young as 10 or 12 already had signs of heart disease.

In the course of the study, a number of children died accidentally or violently, and their hearts and arteries were closely examined at autopsy. Shockingly, the arteries of youngsters whose cholesterol had been elevated had blockages, especially if the children were already smoking, sedentary, and overweight.

This extended the findings from autopsies of young American soldiers killed in battle during the Korean and Vietnam wars. Unlike their contemporaries, Korean and Vietnamese soldiers of similar age, the American soldiers already had clogged arteries.

One in 500 children will be born with genetically elevated cholesterol levels, a condition known as familial hypercholesterolemia. Their arteries quickly clog, CHD develops, and heart attacks occur as early as the teen years and early twenties.

Such children require special attention, beyond just dietary counseling. Ongoing studies at a number of medical centers across the United States have investigated the use of lovastatin (Mevacor) in boys aged 10 to 17 years of age. Lovastatin aggressively slows the body's own liver manufacture of cholesterol. Dosages begin at 10 mg and are increased as needed to 20 mg and then to 40 mg. Cholesterol counts plummet without side effects or problems. The study's authors concluded that using prescription drugs to prevent CHD and heart attacks at a very early age outweighs concerns about the use of these powerful medications.

For most children with higher than normal cholesterol levels, however, the solutions are a matter of lifestyle modification. That means the same low-fat, low-cholesterol, high-fiber diet advocated for adults. Such children should be encouraged to exercise and engage in physical activity rather than spending all their leisure time in front of the TV and computer. And certainly parents must teach them early on about the dangers of cigarette smoking.

Both parents and parents-to-be must make their own lifestyle changes. Kids living with parents who smoke in the home have lower levels of the protective HDL cholesterol and narrower-than-normal coronary arteries. Sadly, such damage persists later in life. And mothers with elevated cholesterol levels themselves tend to give birth to children with damaged arteries.

But what about the safety of placing young children on low-fat diets? Some have voiced concern that growth and development may be impaired. That concern was particularly fueled several years ago after the published report of children who failed to thrive when their parents took diets to extremes, virtually eliminating indispensable fats and many or most of the protein-rich foods.

Subsequent studies have put such fears to rest. The data have been reported in prestigious medical and nutrition journals. A low-fat, low-cholesterol diet, even when given to children during the first three years of life, does not impede physical growth or mental development.

With products available in any supermarket today, kids can still enjoy hot dogs, ice cream, dairy foods of all kinds, luncheon meats, and almost everything else in low-fat, or at least reduced-fat, versions. It's simply a matter of cutting back on saturated fats in animal-based foods and on trans fatty acids in processed foods and fast food. Essentially even the youngest children can follow the same dietary recommendations I propose in this book.

Again, this should be a family affair, with everyone living the same heart-healthy lifestyle including diet and exercise. To rephrase the old adage, your kids are what you eat and how you live. One study presented at a meeting on CHD in the young found (no real surprise) that children whose parents were sedentary and ate impulsively tended to be overweight and sedentary themselves. Habits that extend into adolescence and adulthood are formed during the earliest years of a person's life.

The Teen Years

I know from personal experience that it's more difficult to influence teens than little children. But it's not at all impossible, especially when such influence begins in the early years.

Will teens eat pizzas and burgers even though they know there are healthier choices? Of course. And you don't want to turn your children into neurotics who fear each and every bite of food. But you can expect them to make fatty foods a once-in-a-while treat when out with friends. And you can decide what sorts of foods are available in the house for meals and snacks. Your good example—short of becoming neurotic about it yourself—will do wonders.

At whatever stage of life you begin to improve your children's diet and other behaviors, do it in small steps rather than in one major overnight revolution. Otherwise you will have a counterrevolution on your hands! Take milk as an example. Gradually decrease fat by switching from whole milk to low-fat (2 percent) to lower-fat (1 percent) and then possibly to nonfat skim milk. The same goes for ground beef. Work your way down from regular beef (30 percent fat) to beef with 22 percent fat, then 17 percent, 15 percent, and 10 percent or lower. Your family won't notice the difference, especially in dishes such as chili, spaghetti sauce, lasagna, or Mexican foods like tacos.

Young Adults

Is it really worthwhile to aggressively change your lifestyle? The research speaks for itself. "One in five men between the ages of 30 and 34 has some significant damage to his heart arteries that has probably developed over the past 20 years due to one or more risk factors for heart disease," says Dr. Henry McGill of the Southwest Foundation for Biomedical Research in San Antonio, Texas. He found, again based on autopsy studies, that individuals who had high blood levels of LDL cholesterol were about 2.5 times more likely to have advanced plaque blockages in their coronary arteries than people who did not. His subjects were 760 men and women between the ages of 15 and 34 who had died from an accident, homicide, or suicide. Other studies come to the same conclusion: prevention of heart disease must begin as early as possible.

In my own case, I had my heart attack and first bypass surgery at the tender age of 35. Although I do have a family history, my dad having had a fatal MI at 57, there is no doubt that smoking, poor eating habits, and the resulting high cholesterol, sedentary behavior, and stress all speeded the CHD process. The fact that I am now 58 is all the proof I need that the lifestyle modifications I've followed for the past 17 years, and now suggest to you in this book, really work and can save lives.

Testing cholesterol levels in children remains somewhat controversial. Most authorities agree that children with a family history of very premature heart disease (heart attacks in grandparents and possibly parents earlier than 40) should be tested as toddlers. For those with a history of heart disease in family members younger than 60, tests should be done in early childhood, probably around the sixth birthday. (Not *on* the youngster's birthday, for heaven's sake!)

In the opinion of numerous authorities, all teenagers should have a cholesterol test. Their blood pressure should also be measured. Consider these tests to be crystal balls predicting the future—but this is one time you can change that future in a very positive way.

As a final thought, I believe that all young adults in their twenties should have both cholesterol and blood pressure tested as a routine measure by physicians. For those with normal numbers, tests should be repeated in five years. And for those with abnormalities, this is the time to start making a difference to prevent future CHD.

If we are to end the rule of heart disease as the nation's number one killer, we must begin when heart disease begins: in childhood or as soon as possible.

Heart Disease and the Elderly

Just as it's never too early, it's never too late to start changes to prevent heart disease. Certainly those who have already lived into their sixties, seventies, or more don't have the genes or haven't developed the risk factors that lead to premature CHD, heart attacks, and death. But that doesn't mean it's time to let down your guard.

Of course age itself is a risk factor for heart disease. But even though we can't slow down the chronological aging process—those birthdays just keep on coming—everyone can slow down the process of physiological aging and degeneration.

Make some simple observations of your own. You'll see few, if any, obese, sedentary smokers in the elderly. Conversely, the elderly—including those in their nineties or even 100—have some definite traits in common. They maintain a healthy weight, are nonsmokers, indulge in alcohol moderately, get plenty of physical activity on a regular basis, are generally upbeat and have a zest for life, remain mentally active, tend to think about and help others, and frequently take comfort in their chosen religion. All of us can take a lesson from them—or two or three.

Healthy older men and women also take full advantage of modern medical advances. If they have cholesterol levels or blood pressures that don't respond adequately to lifestyle modifications, they comply with doctors' prescriptions for drugs. And they get annual examinations.

Not surprisingly, research studies provide a scientific foundation for these observations of the elderly. Not too many years ago, most doctors took the rather fatalistic view that there was no reason to try to change the behavior of their older patients. Their rationale ran along the lines that why bother to ask them to change their ways when they don't have that much longer to live anyway. Today we know differently. Making changes and controlling risk factors, even in the oldest men and women, can have a dramatic effect not only on quantity of life, but on quality as well.

I've had the pleasure and privilege to meet and chat with hundreds of elderly men and women during the years following publication of my first book. Asked to do presentations for organizations all over the country, I quickly noticed that audiences had a lot of gray heads. And I learned that older folks make the best possible patients. They follow heart-healthy advice better than practically anyone else—with good reason. The elderly are far more conscious of their own mortality and want to put off the inevitable for as long as possible. They've worked hard all their lives, and now it's time to relax and enjoy the fruits of their labors. But the golden years can be tarnished by poor health and disability. These people know they can make a difference in their own lives.

The statistics regarding heart disease and the elderly are dramatically clear. The best example is an ongoing study conducted by collaborating researchers at medical centers across the country. Nearly 5000 men and women are enrolled. Over a 4.5-year period, doctors learned that in this group aged 60 or older, smokers had a 73 percent greater risk of heart disease than nonsmokers. Diabetics had a 121 percent greater risk. And for every 40-mg elevation in cholesterol levels, risk rose by 20 percent. Conversely, those who followed prescribed treatment and lifestyle changes enjoyed a 27 percent decrease in risk.

In a study termed the Honolulu Heart Program, 2678 men aged 71 to 93 tested the benefits of walking. Risk of first heart attack dropped 15 percent for every additional half-mile a day walked. Those at greatest risk walked less than a quarter-mile, about 2.5 to 3 city blocks, daily. On the other end of the spectrum, those walking at least 1.5 miles a day had the least risk. Many other studies mirror those findings of the benefits of physical activity. And as I discuss in more detail in the exercise chapter, elderly men who remain vigorously active have blood vessels as healthy as men in their twenties. How's that for slowing down the aging clock?

In the old days, doctors figured cholesterol levels were normal at

200 plus a person's age. No more. Now everyone, regardless of age, should get those numbers down to less than 200, and ideally into the 160 to 180 range, with an LDL count of no more than 100. That holds true for both men and women.

The National Institute on Aging conducted a study published in 1995 of 2527 women and 1377 men over 71 years old. They found that those with HDL levels less than 35 were 2.5 times more likely to die as a result of CHD within a one-year period than elderly patients with HDLs over 60. And every milligram increase in HDL lessened risk.

Elevations in total cholesterol are particularly important in elderly women. Those with levels between 200 and 239 had 1.5 times greater risk than women whose numbers were under 200. When cholesterol totals rose above 240, CHD risk doubled.

Diabetes greatly increases the odds of developing CHD for everyone, especially for the elderly. Unfortunately, many older patients are not properly evaluated and diagnosed. No matter one's age, glucose levels should be well under 126. And if the diagnosis of diabetes is made, one can often avoid the need for medication by losing excess weight and doing regular exercise such as walking. Uncontrolled diabetes doubles CHD risk.

While hypertension in which both the upper (systolic) and lower (diastolic) blood pressures is elevated presents more danger of stroke than heart attack, a condition in which the upper number only is high leads to greater CHD risk. Normal blood pressure is less than 130/80. Borderline high is up to 139/89. A reading of 140/90 or more signifies hypertension and should definitely be lowered. Again, lifestyle modifications, including diet and exercise, can often control mild to moderate high blood pressure without having to resort to drugs.

With what we know today, heart disease is largely preventable. Everyone, regardless of age or gender, can and should take preventive measures to avoid this killer.

3
Heart Health in a Nutshell: The Program at a Glance

You and I are really lucky. We're living in a time in history when heart disease is largely preventable. If you've never had a heart attack or bypass surgery, you can be pretty sure you never will: if you make the right decisions about your lifestyle, take the steps necessary to remove risk factors, and work with your doctor to the fullest. And even if you have had a run-in with CHD, you can slash the risks of that ever happening again.

In this chapter I've provided a summary of the steps to take to give yourself a future free of heart disease. Sure, I hope you will read each chapter and follow all my recommendations. But should you want a quick overview at one time or another, this minichapter will serve that purpose.

MOTIVATION AND COMMITMENT

Even if total protection against CHD could be achieved by swallowing one little tablet or capsule, you'd still have to remember to take that pill. Anything in life that's worthwhile takes at least some effort. And when it comes to fighting heart disease, the first step is to make a real commitment.

What's your motivation for protecting your life? For me the list starts with a love for my family that's particularly strong. But that list goes on and on. A great day on the golf course with my buddies. A weekend getaway fishing trip. Beautiful sunsets. Celebrating holidays. Wonderful foods and wines. Looking forward to my grandchildren someday—an experience my own father was cheated out of enjoying.

So, what's your motivation? What will lead you to make the commitment to living a heart-healthy lifestyle? Take a moment to think about your life. Make your own list of reasons to live, and to live well, without disease. Consider all the persons, places, and things on that list as you read this book and make your resolve to follow the program to its fullest.

THE FOUNDATION DIET

Following a heart-healthy diet has never been easier. It is much easier than it was back in the 1980s when I first wrote *The 8-Week Cholesterol Cure*. Many foods that were off-limits then have graduated to the approved list, thanks to new research findings. Here's the diet at a glance.

- The only negative is to cut way back on foods rich in saturated fats (full-fat milk and dairy products, fatty cuts of meat, tropical oils) and trans fat (margarine, commercially baked goods such as cookies and crackers, and fried fast foods).
- Enjoy the healthy fats and oils, limiting them only in terms of total calories to maintain your weight. Those include olive and canola oils, nuts of all sorts, avocados, olives, and manufactured foods made with natural oils rather than hydrogenated fats.
- Have at least two servings of fish, especially fatty fish, weekly. Omega-3 fatty acids from salmon, herring, mackerel, and other fish actually protect against heart disease.
- With those thoughts in mind, forget about counting fat grams.
- Get into the habit of having plenty of fruits and vegetables every day. Start with a minimum of five servings daily, and work yourself up from there. Fresh is best, but canned, dried, and frozen still provide plenty of the nutrients we now know protect the heart. It's easy—even pizza sauce counts!
- Choose whole-grain breads and cereals as often as possible. Limit empty-calorie carbs from white bread, rice, and noodles.
- Forget out-of-date warnings about red meats. Many are full of good nutrition and surprisingly low in fat. Go for pork loin, tenderloin, and ham. Choose cuts of beef with the word *loin* or *round* in their names. Discover a whole new world of special breeds of cattle providing beef cuts of all sorts with no more fat than skinless chicken breast.
- Think soluble fiber—that special kind found in oats, beans, barley, prunes, and many other foods. Soluble fiber actually removes cholesterol from your bloodstream.
- Get plenty of fluids. Not just water. Drink juice, nonfat or lowfat milk, and other beverages liberally throughout the day.

- Really *enjoy* your foods. Take the time to taste each and every bite. Don't rush meals or gobble foods while doing other things. Smell and taste those foods slowly, swallowing before you take another bite.
- If you enjoy alcoholic beverages, do so in moderation. One or two drinks daily for men, one for women, actually offer protection against heart disease.

EXERCISE AND PHYSICAL ACTIVITY

Centuries ago, Hippocrates wrote, in effect although in loftier language, "Use it or lose it." No need to go to the gym unless that's what you prefer, but get active on a regular basis. Enjoy your physical activities: dancing, gardening, walking, bicycling, swimming—whatever you like. Start because you know you should. When you see how good you feel, you won't want to stop!

For optimum heart health, shoot for a total of 15 miles per week. That's about 2 miles of daily walking or its equivalent. You needn't do it all at once; exercise "points" add up throughout the day.

TESTING YOUR HEART'S HEALTH

No single risk factor is responsible for the development and progression of heart disease. Over the years we have learned that many such factors come into play. And we can measure our risk with a variety of tests that every man and woman should have done in his or her doctor's office. Here's what your physician can learn from a small sample of your blood.

- *The lipid profile.* This includes your total cholesterol, the "bad" LDL cholesterol, the "good" HDL cholesterol, and triglycerides. From these numbers, one can calculate a risk ratio. Avoid all foods and beverages other than water for 12 to 14 hours prior to the testing.
- *Other influences.* Excessive levels of the amino acid homocysteine increase the likelihood of plaque formation in the arteries. Both high and low amounts of the blood sugar glucose raise your risk. Uric acid not only leads to a painful condition called gout but also puts you at increased CHD risk. Thyroid hormone, produced by a gland in your neck, can decrease with age, making you more likely to gain weight, have reduced energy and stamina, and develop heart disease.

■ *The "baddest" bad cholesterol.* Those with a family history of heart disease, especially, should know about lipoprotein (a), or Lp(a) (pronounced "el-pee-little-a"). This nasty form of LDL cholesterol can put you at risk even when other factors are perfectly normal. That's the bad news. The good news is we can control Lp(a).

■ *Blood pressure.* You'll also want your doctor to test your blood pressure. Even slight elevations of the systolic (top number) and diastolic (bottom number) place you at greater risk of heart attack and stroke. Mild to moderate hypertension responds beautifully to lifestyle modifications, often obviating the need for medications.

■ *Cardiac inflammation.* For many years, doctors felt that blockage of the arteries began as an effort of the body to heal an injury to the endothelial lining of those arteries. Something has to initiate the process, which is facilitated by excessive cholesterol, triglycerides, and other blood factors. Now there's compelling scientific evidence that heart disease may be instigated by an inflammation of some sort. At the very least, inflammation may be a marker or indication that heart disease exists and is progressing. What causes the inflammation? No one knows for sure. The notion that it may be a response to a viral or bacterial infection has gotten mixed reviews. This will continue to be an arena of intense investigation in the years to come.

In the meantime, however, we can all use the existing knowledge that inflammation is somehow involved. First, we can test whether inflammation exists in our hearts. That's done through a test called hs-CRP, which measures the specific inflammation marker C-reactive protein. The normal range is 0.7 to 1.1. mg/dL.

What can be done if the test detects inflammation by way of elevated CRP? Some believe that the recommendation of one aspirin tablet daily, already known to reduce clot formation, may reduce inflammation. In fact, CRP does not predict risk for those taking daily aspirin. And if CRP is indeed in the high range, you must be particularly aggressive in modifying the risk factors that can be controlled. That means getting cholesterol levels way down, reducing blood pressure, and so forth.

SUPPLEMENTS YOUR HEART WILL THANK YOU FOR

Yes, you'll want to make some dietary improvements, but well-chosen supplements can boost the nutrients your heart needs for optimum health.

- *Antioxidants.* Years of research at the world's most prestigious medical centers has shown unequivocally that the oxidized form of LDL cholesterol does the most damage. Stop that oxidation with the antioxidant vitamin E (400 to 800 IUs), vitamin C (1000 mg), beta-carotene (6 mg), and selenium (200 μg). As a bonus, those antioxidants also keep the lining of the arteries, the endothelium, healthy and flexible.
- *Niacin.* Eighty percent of the cholesterol in your blood is produced by your liver; diet accounts for only 20 percent, at most. Niacin, also known as vitamin B_3 and nicotinic acid, stops the body's excess production. But it does much more: It raises the good HDL cholesterol, slashes triglycerides, and controls newly discovered independent risk factors, including Lp(a) and small, dense LDL.
- *B vitamins.* To B or not to B is no longer the question. We know now that we can completely control buildup of the amino acid homocysteine with daily supplementation of three B vitamins: B_6 (2 mg), B_{12} (6 μg), and folic acid (400 to 800 μg). Some researchers believe that homocysteine elevations are as dangerous as high cholesterol levels.
- *Minerals.* We hear a lot about restricting sodium to reduce or prevent hypertension. But sodium is just one of the minerals that influence blood pressure. Rather than simply cutting back on sodium, we should make an effort to increase our intake of the minerals that research has shown to lower blood pressure. Those include magnesium, calcium, and potassium. Shoot for 300 mg of magnesium and at least 800 mg of calcium daily; most diets don't provide that much, so supplements will probably be needed. There are, however, plenty of dietary sources of potassium; and salt substitutes replace sodium with potassium.
- *Phytosterols.* It almost sounds too good to be true, but we can actually *block* the cholesterol in foods from getting into the bloodstream. Literally hundreds of research studies document the ability of phytosterols (plant sterols) to block the absorp-

tion of cholesterol. And regular intake can result in about a 10 percent cholesterol reduction in your blood.

- *Pantethine.* This derivative of pantothenic acid can dramatically raise HDL and lower triglycerides.
- *Fish oils.* All of us should eat fish, especially fatty fish, at least twice a week. The omega-3 fatty acids found in fish reduce formations of blood clots and lower triglycerides. But if you just don't like fish, supplement your diet with at least 1000 mg (1 gram) of fish oil per day.

WHAT'S HOT AND WHAT'S NOT

We can do a lot to protect ourselves from heart disease. Some things really work, while others merely pad the bank accounts of those promoting the product or service.

- *Aspirin.* The vast majority of men and women would profit by simply taking a single tablet of ordinary aspirin daily. Check with your doctor as to the best dosage. The American Heart Association recommends one 81-mg children's aspirin tablet daily, with a twice-monthly booster of a full-strength 325-mg tablet. Others, including myself, believe that as long as you can tolerate it, the larger dose may be more effective in preventing clot formation and in reducing inflammation.
- *Statin drugs.* Prescription-only drugs called HMG co-A reductase inhibitors, commonly termed "statins," limit production of cholesterol by the liver. Of these, atorvastatin (Lipitor) is the most potent, though not everyone needs that level of potency to achieve optimal reductions. Solid research documents the combination of statins, specifically simvastatin (Zocor) at 10 mg, with 1500 to 3000 mg of regular-release niacin.
- *Cholestin.* Urged by the major pharmaceutical manufacturers of statin drugs, the FDA has tried to stop sales of an over-the-counter cholesterol-lowering agent called Cholestin. This natural substance is derived from yeast grown on red rice; it has been used in Chinese medicine and cooking for decades. Why the fuss? Because Cholestin is a naturally occurring, though lower potency, statin. It really works, providing at least a 10 percent reduction.
- *Guggulipid.* Used for decades, if not centuries, by healers in India, this plant-derived substance does have a cholesterol-

lowering effect. Unfortunately, little research has been done and proper dosage is uncertain.

■ *Garlic.*   Ignore those radio and television ads promoting garlic supplements. Research indicates very little cholesterol reduction, if any at all. Save your money. Instead, cook with garlic if you like it since garlic as food rather than supplement may have additional antioxidant benefits.

■ *Soy foods and supplements.*   The FDA has given its approval for companies to make heart-health claims for soy products. Research shows benefit from consuming 25 grams of soy protein daily. But to get the benefits, soy must be consumed each and every day. Whole foods are better than supplements.

■ *Co-Q10.*   The full name of this supplement is coenzyme Q10. Its chemical term is ubiquinone, alluding to the fact that it is ubiquitous, meaning everywhere, in the body's cells and tissues. It has absolutely no cholesterol benefits. Although earlier research showed some potential benefit for those suffering from heart failure, current findings indicate no benefit at all.

■ *Chelation therapy.*   This is flat-out quackery. The substance EDTA, given by a nurse in a doctor's office or clinic, in a series of expensive fusions, is said to bind onto (chelate) calcium in arterial plaque. This has been debunked by every *legitimate* research study, although practitioners come up with useless, nonscientific results and testimonials from satisfied customers. Benefits are most likely due to the placebo effect and lifestyle modifications urged by the "caring" support staff.

■ *Extra-corporeal counter pulsation.*   There is absolutely no scientific validity that this heavily advertised therapy, ECCP, can result in regression of atherosclerosis. Promoters base its effectiveness on a completely false premise. Just because this treatment is offered by licensed physicians doesn't mean it works. It does not.

WEIGHT MANAGEMENT

The problem with going on a diet is that almost everyone will go off that diet. The only thing that really works is your personal decision to make permanent changes in your eating patterns and physical activity. Sorry, there are no miracles here. But there are approaches that help.

- Keep a daily log of what you eat and drink and when you do so. Learn what foods are most likely contributing excessive calories, and figure out how to eliminate them.
- Avoid or completely eliminate the carbohydrate foods that provide virtually no nutrition and nothing but lots of calories: white breads, noodles, rice, white potatoes, and sugars and desserts.
- "Spoil" your appetite by eating a small snack, perhaps a piece of fruit, about 20 minutes prior to major meals. This will boost your blood sugar (glucose) level so you are not "starving" when you sit down to eat.
- Don't eat while doing something else. Concentrate on the foods you're eating and enjoy the taste. Eat more slowly, chewing and swallowing each mouthful before taking another bite.
- Increase physical activity as much as possible. Take a walk for 10 minutes in lieu of a coffee-and-doughnut break.
- Cut way back on alcohol. It's not just a matter of calories. A drink tends to relax inhibitions and make you more vulnerable to increased food intake.

THE MIND-BODY-HEART CONNECTION

I began this little summary with the thought that life is, indeed, worth living. But stress, depression, and other mental strain can undermine our enjoyment of our lives. And there's no doubt that those factors, while not as easy to measure as blood pressure or cholesterol, have a horribly adverse effect on our hearts.

Not for a moment do I have the brazen audacity to tell you that I have all the answers and solutions for coping with your own situation. But here are a few thoughts to consider.

- Try being a little nicer to yourself. Give yourself a bit of priority, rather than always playing second fiddle to your family and work.
- Make a deliberate effort to be nicer to strangers. Put a quarter into a parking meter that's about to expire. Open a door for someone. Just smile at a person you pass on the street.
- Compose a list of things that are bothering you and see if there aren't some ways to confront and deal with them.
- Seek the support of others. Maybe there's a member of the

clergy or a friend you feel you could trust in conversation about what's troubling you.

■ Don't hesitate to seek professional help. Your physician might recommend some temporary medications, or possibly a counselor. Often just a few sessions can provide tremendous benefit. There's absolutely no reason to feel any sense of shame in admitting you need some help.

■ A bright outlook on life supports our resolve to do the right things to protect our hearts' health. Conversely, a dark mental state can undermine our best intentions and lead us to harmful behaviors. A happy heart is a healthy heart!

KEEP UP TO DATE ON HEART HEALTH INFORMATION

I hate to admit this, but every single book is at least somewhat obsolete by the time it hits the store shelves. Yes, even this one. Though I've made every effort to make last-minute additions and changes right up to the time of publication, the march of progress never stops.

So here's my offer and promise to you. I will review all the medical and scientific journals every week, attend important medical meetings, scour the professional Web sites on the Internet, and discuss the latest developments in research with my contacts across the country and around the world. I'll check out new foods, new health products and treatments, and various controversial issues. And I'll summarize that information on a quarterly basis in my publication *The Diet-Heart Newsletter*. You'll be as up to date as your doctors, maybe more so, and you'll be in the best possible position to keep your heart healthy.

Some of the readers of my first book back in 1987 have subscribed to the newsletter since the very first issue that same year. Many physicians subscribe and they tell me that my newsletter is the best review of the latest developments on the market. I also answer all my readers' questions.

Please feel free to take a few minutes to send me a self-addressed, stamped, business-size envelope. I'll send you a free sample issue along with subscription information. The address is:

The Diet-Heart Newsletter
PO Box 2039
Venice, CA 90294

4

Good Food, Good Times, Good Health

To me, this is the most exciting section of the book. Who doesn't love food? I know I do, and that's why I'm so happy to report that following a heart-healthy diet is no longer the complicated, difficult matter it once was. Today there's no reason to count every gram of fat or give up the foods you enjoy. In fact, if you were to come to my house for a visit, you might be shocked to see my family eating steak, meatloaf, rich caesar salads, eggs for breakfast, and luscious custards for dessert.

Actually, I wince a bit when I look at the cover of the original book offering readers cholesterol reduction "without deprivation." In retrospect, the diet I ate and recommended back then was, indeed, deprivation. But there have been dramatic changes in thinking since those days, thanks to new research investigations.

We should view food as a blessing, not something to condemn or feel guilty about. You won't get any finger-wagging here, no scare tactics. Instead of branding this food or that as "death on a plate" or "food porn," as others do, I want to stress the positive with a cornucopia of delicious, healthy foods to be thoroughly enjoyed.

Most countries issue dietary guidelines for their people, emphasizing those foods that contribute to good health. The United States has its own recommendations, most notably utilizing the Food Pyramid to illustrate priorities in food choices. Rather remarkably, however, the good advice to "enjoy your food" is conspicuously absent from the U.S. guidelines. Virtually every other country counsels its citizens to do so, often in flowing, almost poetic fashion.

Americans really need that advice. Too many don't take the time to really savor their food. This is the country that coined the phrase "fast food." We gulp it down without tasting it, emphasizing quantity rather than quality. This "chow down" attitude leads, in large part, to the current epidemic of obesity in the United States. The food industry, for the most part, fuels the problem by making and advertising foods that are high in calories, fat, sugar, and salt.

Modern stresses make matters worse. As a nation, we gobble sugary breakfast cereals to start the day. Lunch consists of fried stuff that's almost unrecognizable under layers of breading. And by the end of the day, we're so totally stressed out that we practically anesthetize ourselves with a nonstop orgy of feeding that starts at dinner and ends only when the lights finally go out for the night. All without really tasting or thinking about the food we've consumed.

We need to stop and smell and savor our food. Think about each delicious bite. Chew and swallow every forkful before shoving in another load. Concentrate on the food and, ideally, some pleasant conversation rather than the television.

Does the relatively simple lifestyle change of improving one's diet really make a difference? The answer is more than a matter of opinion. Today we have the unequivocal proof.

Doctors at the Harvard School of Public Health looked at data from 44,875 men aged 40 to 75 years for eight years. When the Physicans' Health Study began in 1986, no one in the group had either cancer or cardiovascular disease. By way of questionnaires, the men were divided into two groups. One consumed what might be called the "prudent diet," including plenty of fruits and vegetables, whole grains, fish and poultry, low-fat dairy, and beans and legumes. The second group followed a Western pattern, characterized by a high intake of red meat, refined grains, processed meats, sweets, desserts, fried foods, and high-fat dairy products.

During the course of the study, 1089 men suffered both fatal and nonfatal heart attacks. Which group did better? First the scientists statistically teased out risk factors such as smoking, blood pressure, and such, to level the playing field so that the only difference between the two groups was their food choices. Then they assigned the number 1.0 as average risk of suffering a cardiovascular event.

Men in the prudent diet group had a risk of 1.0, 0.87, 0.79, 0.75, and 0.70, depending on how heart-healthy each of the five subgroups was. Conversely, the Western diet group, divided into five similar subgroups, had risk levels of 1.0, 1.21, 1.36, 1.40, and 1.64.

As we'll see throughout this book, research studies have examined both food patterns and specific foods very closely during the past several years. Some of the conclusions have been predictable: avoid fatty, processed foods. Others have been pleasantly surprising: don't worry so much about total fat; make a point of seeking out certain healthy fats; and enjoy a wide variety of foods that will provide the previously overlooked nutrients that can protect against heart disease.

Rather coincidentally, while I was working on this book, the American Heart Association issued a completely revised version of its own dietary guidelines. I'm happy to say that the AHA guidelines and my own recommendations are very much in tune with each other.

The first emphasis was placed on consuming a wide variety of foods containing plenty of fruits, vegetables, and whole grains. Rather than stressing total fat consumption, which should not exceed 30 percent of calories as fat, the AHA recommended avoidance of saturated fats and trans fatty acids from processed oils. Rather surprisingly, they warned that an ultra-low-fat diet such as that advocated by Pritikin and Ornish may do more harm than good. In fact, the AHA pointed to the benefits of healthy oils and advised the public to consume fish—especially fatty fish, which contain the healthful omega-3 fatty acids—at least twice weekly. And they recognized the value of adding plant sterols, which block the absorption of dietary cholesterol, by way of supplements and margarines.

By practical necessity, the AHA guidelines were just that: guidelines rather than specific recommendations. In the coming pages you will learn how to make practical food choices.

Much has been written about the so-called French paradox: Perhaps the red wine does contribute to health—we'll discuss that in the coming pages. Maybe the French are genetically capable of metabolizing cream and butter sauces without clogging their arteries. But there are other realities as well.

The French croissant is perhaps a third of the size of those baked here. Serving sizes of those rich dishes are actually tiny. Fresh fruits and vegetables constitute a huge percentage of the diet. And the average French man and woman dwell on the presentation, aroma, and exquisite taste of each and every dish. Bottom line: the French actually eat a lot less fat and a lot fewer calories than we think they do.

With that in mind, I've decided to break down my thoughts and recommendations—and a lot of wonderful surprises—into a series of bite-sized sections. The menu will include courses on fats, red meats, alcohol, sugar, coffee and tea, seafood, fruits and vegetables, grains and carbohydrate foods, and even how you can eat cholesterol-rich foods like whole eggs without doing your arteries any harm at all. So sit back, read, and enjoy.

MOM WAS RIGHT: EAT YOUR FRUITS AND VEGETABLES (AND DON'T FORGET THE GRAINS AND BEANS)

Okay, let's get one thing straight right off the bat. I am not now, nor have I ever been or plan to be, a vegetarian. I love food way too much to give up the incredible variety of meats, fish and seafood, and dairy products. Moreover, while vegetarians are no doubt healthy, it's probably not what they *don't* eat, but, rather, what they *do* eat. That means plenty of fruits, vegetables, grains and cereals, and beans and nuts.

These foods are loaded with nutrients, fiber, antioxidants more complete than you can get from a bottle, and stuff they probably haven't discovered yet. Think I'm kidding about that last one? Everyone has heard of beta-carotene, but did you know that it is just one of nearly 500 carotenoids found in a carrot? Why settle for one when you can get 500? Besides, almost all plant foods are extremely low in fat and have no cholesterol whatsoever.

Sure, nuts, olives, and avocados have a lot of fat. But that fat happens to be good for us. It doesn't "count" in a heart-healthy diet.

Because I'm so involved with all things having to do with heart health, reading the scientific and medical journals religiously and attending scientific meetings and seminars every year, I'm tempted to cite study after study to prove my point. But I'll restrain myself and give you just a brief overview of the evidence for giving foods from the plant kingdom a prominent place in your diet. (For those who wish to pursue the subject more, see the references at the end of this book.)

- Doctors at Stanford University found that while a typical low-fat, low-cholesterol diet works, a similar diet with more added veggies and grains works twice as well. One group of subjects ate the typical heart-healthy diet. After four weeks, total cholesterol dropped by 9.2 mg on average, with LDL going down by 7.0 mg. Those eating the diet with added grains and veggies achieved a 17.6 mg drop in total cholesterol, and LDL fell by 13.8 mg.
- Two studies at Harvard University, published in October 2000, demonstrated that a higher intake of plant foods produced a dramatic drop in the risk of CHD for both men and women. Women consuming the most plant food, though they were not vegetarians, had the lowest risk of suffering heart attacks— 70 percent lower than average. Those eating the fewest plant foods and the most foods high in saturated fat had 64 percent more heart attacks than average. Subjects were part of the

long-term Nurses' Health Study. Findings were similar for men enrolled in the counterpart Physicians' Health Study.

- A year earlier, in 1999, investigators showed that the more fruits and vegetables a group of men and women ate, the lower their risk of having a stroke. For some reason, certain vegetables—leafy greens, broccoli, brussels sprouts—and citrus fruits and juices offered the most protection.

- A major study called DASH (Dietary Approaches to Stop Hypertension) found that a diet rich in fruits, vegetables, and low-fat animal foods substantially lowered blood pressure. How much? In those with mild to moderate hypertension, about the same as could be expected from medications.

- Some investigations have shown a link between protection against heart disease and antioxidant levels in those consuming lots of fruits and veggies. Others point to the influence of fiber from a diet rich in fruits, vegetables, and cereals. Whatever the principal "active ingredient"—and there is probably more than one—there has *never* been a single study that failed to demonstrate the almost amazing protective powers of plant foods.

Variety Is the Spice of Life

Broccoli is good for you. So are bananas and blueberries. Cooked tomatoes appear to work better than raw ones. Although fruits and vegetables have a lot of nutritional goodies in common, each appears to have a particular benefit. So the trick seems to be to eat as many different kinds as possible.

We've seen how leafy greens and broccoli protect against stroke. The antioxidant lycopene in cooked tomato foods, such as juice, ketchup, pizza, and pasta sauces, helps to break down bad LDL cholesterol and appears to inhibit its production by the liver.

Purple grape juice contains the same flavonoids that are thought to give red wine its protective qualities. Grape juice improves the ability of the arteries to dilate, thus increasing blood flow. And it reduces the oxidation of LDL in the blood (oxidized LDL does the most damage in the arteries).

Red wine also provides a rich source of substances called polyphenols, which act as antioxidants and protect the lining, or endothelium, of the arteries. Some say that's the reason for the "French paradox" by which people there are protected against heart disease. But not everyone likes red wine, and others drink no alcoholic beverages at all. Yet everyone can benefit from the grape's polyphenols by way of grape seed extract tablets.

Four tablets of grape seed extract (200 mg) provide the equivalent of one four-ounce glass of red wine. On the ORAC scale of antioxidant efficiency, which I'll get to in a moment, grape seed extract absolutely soars. Moreover, the polyphenols of those tablets work with vitamins C and E to maintain a higher level of those antioxidants in the blood over time.

Not all grape seed extract tablets are created equal. Look for one of the several brands that list Mega-Natural extract, shown to be of the highest purity and potency. Such products are not a replacement for fruits and vegetables, but they can boost your level of protection. For further information, you can visit the website www.polyphenolics.com.

Ounce for ounce, prunes pack the most antioxidants of all fruits and keep LDL cholesterol from getting nasty. And bananas, Americans' favorite fruit, are loaded with the mineral potassium, which helps keep blood pressure in check.

The next time you're in the supermarket, consider shopping by the colors. The very same plant substances that give fruits and vegetables their marvelous spectrum of colors provide a similar variety of heart-protecting antioxidants, bioflavonoids, and polyphenols. Paint your heart healthy with blue from blueberries, green from leafy vegetables, orange from citrus, red from grapes, and so on.

The experts at the Human Nutrition Research Center on Aging at Tufts University in Boston have come up with a way to measure the antioxidant potential of foods to protect against CHD and other degenerative diseases. Their system is termed ORAC, which stands for oxygen radical absorbance capacity.

The top antioxidant foods, based on ORAC units per 3.5-ounce (100-gram) serving, are:

Prunes	5770	Broccoli	890
Raisins	2830	Beets	840
Blueberries	2400	Oranges	750
Kale	1770	Red grapes	739
Spinach	1260	Cherries	670
Brussels sprouts	980	Onions	450
Plums	949	Corn	400

The more of these high-ORAC foods you eat, the more antioxidants build up in your bloodstream, protecting you against free radicals, the type of oxygen that damages tissues and organs.

Five or More Servings: Easier Than You Think

In Japan, dietary guidelines call for eating at least 23 different foods each and every day. At first glance, that might seem like an impossible goal. But the Japanese typically eat small, even tiny, servings of a wide variety of foods at any given meal. And many dishes, such as sukiyaki, a type of vegetable soup-stew with a little chicken or fish, contain easily a dozen ingredients.

Many Western dishes similarly combine a whole roster of vegetables. Salads include various greens, as well as tomatoes, radishes, shredded carrots, sliced beets, and on and on. Think about how you pile your platter high with interesting combinations when you visit a buffet-style restaurant. Do the same at home by keeping little canisters of ingredients in your refrigerator. The stews that taste best are those with many vegetables, including onions, turnips, rutabaga, sweet potatoes, celery, and other root vegetables you probably wouldn't eat alone. The same goes for vegetable soups of all kinds.

I'm sure that boiled or steamed vegetables are very good for you, but they can quickly get boring. Get out of the rut. Try sautéing asparagus with some extra-virgin olive oil and a sprinkle of tarragon and thyme. Roast tomato halves topped with grated parmesan cheese. Microwave acorn squash with a little brown sugar or maple syrup. Mash nutrient-rich sweet potatoes instead of white potatoes. Cut bananas lengthwise, then fry them and serve with black beans and rice along with chicken in the Caribbean fashion. Sauté broccoli and carrots and then add a bit of Chinese black bean sauce. Roast a casserole dish of winter root vegetables with some olive oil and fresh herbs.

One of the most successful ways I found to get my kids to eat more fruits when they were little was to prepare fruit platters. When Ross and Jenny came home from school, I'd slice some apples and make faces with raisins. Or I'd fashion a plate of finger-sized fruits with a dipping bowl of fruit-flavored yogurt. The kids and their friends would devour those platters in a few minutes. Yet if someone offered them a bowl of unpeeled apples, oranges, and bananas, they'd turn it down.

Most people—quite rightly—roll their eyes at the suggestion of carrot sticks and celery as a replacement snack for potato chips or candy. Boring. How about an apple while watching TV? Still boring. But make that a taffy apple crusted with nuts, and it's a different story. Just a few extra calories and a few grams of fat and you've given yourself another serving of fruit for the day. Or slice a pear or a banana and drizzle some chocolate syrup over it. Cut the scoop of ice cream you're planning to eat in half and fill out the bowl with fresh berries. For an adult dessert or snack, try peeled orange slices with a splash of Meyer's dark rum.

Still, you say, at least five servings a day? Preferably seven or even nine? How can you possibly eat that much food? Well, the answer is that it's not as much food as you think. It comes down to the size of a serving, which, especially in the United States, is a lot less than people typically guess.

A serving of cooked vegetables or vegetable juice is ½ cup (4 ounces). For raw vegetables, it's 1 cup (8 ounces). For the next few days, make it a point to measure out your vegetables and juices. I'm confident that what you've been calling one serving is actually two, or even three.

The same holds for fruit. A serving of any fruit juice is 1 cup (8 ounces). Glance through Table 1 for listings of fresh, frozen, and canned fruit as well as dried fruit. Two little figs constitute a serving. How many do you eat at once? A serving of honeydew melon is one-eighth of a melon, not one-quarter. Just 2 tablespoons of raisins make a serving.

So you see, those five, seven, nine, or even more servings of fruits and vegetables daily aren't that big a deal. Let's take a look at how you might work them into a typical day.

For breakfast you might start with a glass of juice. That might be 4 ounces of carrot, tomato, or V-8 juice or an 8-ounce glass of any fruit juice. Then slice a half banana into your cereal, or add ¾ cup of blueberries.

Table 1. SERVING SIZES OF FRUIT

Fresh, Frozen, and Unsweetened Canned Fruit	
Apple	1
Applesauce	½ cup
Apricot	4
Banana	½
Blackberries	¾ cup
Blueberries	¾ cup
Cantaloupe	⅓ cup
Cherries	12 fresh; ½ cup canned
Fig	2
Fruit cocktail	½ cup
Grapefruit	½ medium; ¾ cup segments
Grapes	15
Honeydew melon	⅛
Kiwi	1 large
Mandarin orange	¾ cup segments
Mango	½ small
Nectarine	1 medium
Orange	1 medium
Papaya	1 cup cubed
Peach	1 medium; ¾ cup canned
Pear	1 small; ½ cup, 2 halves canned

Fresh, Frozen, and Unsweetened Canned Fruit

Persimmon	2
Pineapple	¾ cup cubed; ⅓ cup canned
Plum	2
Pomegranate	½
Raspberries	1 cup
Strawberries	1¼ cup
Tangerine	2
Watermelon	1¼ cubes

Dried Fruit

Apples	4 rings
Apricots	7 halves
Dates	2½ medium
Figs	1½
Prunes	3 medium
Raisins	2 tbsp

At your midmorning and midafternoon break, try to replace the coffee and doughnut with a glass of juice or a piece of fruit—at least two or three days a week. Try it for a while, and you might find such snacks are actually far more satisfying.

Most of us are far too busy to do much in the way of preparing lunch. And without planning, that can mean urgent hunger that's satisfied with high-calorie, high-fat, low-nutrient fast food. Here's a suggestion for something even faster: soup. A nice steaming bowl is extremely satisfying and remarkably soothing at midday. Chicken and vegetable, minestrone, lentil, split pea, beef and barley, the list goes on. Either order a bowl at a restaurant or heat up a container you bring from home in a microwave. You'll get two or three servings of veggies in that one meal.

Keep some dried fruit at work. Perhaps little snack boxes of raisins. Or a pop-top can of applesauce or diced peaches. That sure beats running to the candy machine.

For the evening meal, get into the habit of putting two or three different vegetables on the plate. Start the meal with a nice salad—not just iceberg lettuce. And I've already made some suggestions for desserts and evening snacks.

If you actually did all the things I've recommended, you'd tally up nine or more servings daily. Some days more, some days less. Soon it becomes a way of life. Your heart will thank you for it.

FATS: THE GOOD, THE BAD, AND THE UGLY

The story of how medical authorities now view fats and oils in the diet is a great example of how the research process develops. When doctors first made the observation that men participating in the Framingham Heart Study who ate more fat suffered more heart attacks, the conclusion was that the total amount of fat, along with cholesterol, should be reduced.

The American Heart Association, and then the National Cholesterol Education Program and others, began to recommend a diet that had, at most, 30 percent of its calories as fat. That fat was to be divided, more or less equally, as saturated, monounsaturated, and polyunsaturated. I took that a step further, recommending a maximum of 20 percent fat. And some, including Nathan Pritikin and later Dr. Dean Ornish, went to the extreme of virtually eliminating all fat and all dairy foods. Counting those fat grams was complicated.

But, as is always the case, the research effort continued. One study after another revealed that the real villain was saturated fat. In fact, those consuming large amounts of fat in the form of healthy oils were actually at *less* risk of CHD than those following an ultra-low-fat, practically vegetarian diet.

We'll get around to sorting out the details of all the different kinds of fats and oils, and their component parts, the fatty acids, in the coming pages. But first, recognize that there are only three sources of calories available to you: fat, protein, and carbohydrates. If you cut back on one, you have to increase another in order to keep caloric intake equal.

Thus the typical prescription for a heart-healthy diet meant cutting back on fat and eating more carbohydrates, preferably in the form of whole grains and cereals, fruits, and vegetables. On the face of it, that sounds pretty good. But the results were not exactly as planned.

Yes, total and LDL cholesterol fell. That was good. But the protective HDL also came down, and triglycerides rose. In the beginning, authorities simply accepted that trade-off, believing that HDL and triglycerides were not as important as total and LDL cholesterol. Then more data came in.

It gradually became evident that the risk ratio of total cholesterol and LDL to HDL cholesterol was a more accurate predictor of heart disease than total cholesterol and LDL alone. As the HDL declines, that risk ratio worsens. Even with reductions in total and LDL cholesterol, reducing total fat intake often resulted in actually increasing one's CHD risk.

And then there was the issue of triglycerides. For years doctors assumed that these fat particles in the blood were more or less innocuous. They became concerned only when triglycerides exceeded 500 mg/dL, more in fear of damage to the pancreas than to the arteries.

Again, research data contradicted that common belief. It became more and more apparent that high levels of triglycerides, especially in combination with a lowered level of HDL, constituted a risk factor independent of total and LDL cholesterol. Those following a very-low-fat, high-carbohydrate diet were actually trading one CHD risk for another.

Even in my earliest writings, I recognized that certain fats should not count. Oats, for example, have the highest fat content of all the cereal grains, yet consuming them is a heart-healthy thing to do. And fish, though frequently as high in fat as prime beef, actually protects the heart. But I, too, advocated a low-fat approach to the diet for many years.

Gradually, I began to change my tune. First came the revelations that the so-called Mediterranean diet could be as protective as the low-fat, AHA-recommended diet. The Mediterranean diet racked up 30 percent or even more of its calories from fat, but that fat came from olive oil, olives, nuts, and fish.

Closer to home, researchers at Loma Linda University in California observed that those who ate a lot of nuts as part of their daily diets improved their cholesterol counts and slashed their risk of heart disease. The finding held true for peanuts, walnuts, and almonds in separate studies. Was it just a matter of nuts replacing the animal fats in meats? No, study subjects were Seventh Day Adventists who followed a lacto-ovo-vegetarian diet, that is, a vegetarian diet that includes dairy products and eggs. Having eaten lunch at the university's cafeteria, I can testify that such a diet contains a lot of saturated fat. So the fats in the nuts somehow conferred CHD protection.

In the meantime, the benefits of omega-3 fatty acids, a type of polyunsaturated fat found in fish and, to a lesser extent, flaxseed, appeared in an avalanche of research findings. Not only did the fish oil raise HDL and lower triglycerides, but it also lessened the likelihood of blood clots forming, improved blood pressure, and seemed to control some types of heart rhythm disturbances. The data were so compelling it almost sounded a cure-all too good to believe.

Finally, practically every week I was reading new articles in scientific and medical journals documenting the protective qualities of various oils: olive oil, canola oil, grapeseed oil. All appeared to confer CHD protection beyond simply replacing saturated fats.

The big concern with the liberal use of nuts, oils, and other fatty foods, which add even more calories to the diet, is that the already horrible problem of obesity might worsen. It's like the dilemma presented by alcohol: moderate use can slash CHD risk, but recommending alcohol to the population at large might well lead to alcoholism and the problems associated with drunkenness.

Here's a good example of how oils might increase caloric intake. It's become rather fashionable, especially in Italian restaurants, to offer cruets of extra-virgin olive oil for bread dipping. But wouldn't that practice add calories as compared with eating the bread plain? Researchers put the question to the test. In a restaurant setting they gave some diners bread alone while others also received olive oil. Then they measured the total amount eaten and calculated the calories. Surprise! The oil dippers actually ate less and consumed fewer calories, not more. It appears that the bread dipped in oil is more satisfying. Diners didn't simply eat and eat and eat as they might with the less satisfying plain bread. And since olive oil has no more effect on cholesterol levels than plain bread, the bottom line was that we are better off enjoying the wonderful flavor of bread dipped in rich, satisfying extra-virgin olive oil than stoically eating bread alone.

As I reported more and more such data in my newsletter, readers wrote scathing letters to me saying I was sabotaging heart-healthy diets. Some even feared for me, arguing that if I followed my own advice regarding a more liberal view of diet, I would wind up having another bypass surgery!

But I wasn't totally alone. I was delighted when, in 1998, the American Heart Association published a statement in its official journal, *Circulation,* advising against very-low-fat diets that contained no more than 15 percent of calories from fat. Nathan Pritikin had advocated a 10 percent fat diet, while Dr. Dean Ornish recommended a near-vegetarian diet with no added oil whatsoever and no fish—not something many people wanted to follow anyway. For most men and women, such radical diets do more harm than good, the AHA proclaimed.

Then in October 2000, the AHA went a giant step further. Its completely revised dietary guidelines no longer spoke of specific numbers, such as 30 percent of calories from fat. Rather than telling the population to avoid or eliminate certain foods, the AHA took the positive stance of emphasizing healthy foods that would, of necessity, crowd out foods containing large amounts of saturated fats. Amen.

Here, in a nutshell, are the AHA's dietary guidelines:

- Choose an overall balanced diet with a wide variety of foods from all major food groups. Emphasize at least five daily servings of fruits and vegetables and at least six servings of grain products, including whole grains.
- Include fat-free and low-fat dairy products, fish, legumes, poultry, and lean meats. Eat at least two servings of fish per week.
- Limit foods high in saturated fats and cholesterol, consuming no more than 300 mg of cholesterol for most people, and no more than 200 mg for those with heart disease or other risk factors.
- Limit trans fatty acids found in foods containing partially hydrogenated vegetable oils such as cookies, crackers, and baked goods, commercially fried foods, and certain margarines.

This book, of course, goes into far greater detail on how to most efficiently—and most deliciously—achieve those goals. And there are some guidelines such as strict salt and sodium restriction with which I and many other authorities do not agree. You'll find the specifics elsewhere in the book.

Zeroing in on the Good Fats

For decades, epidemiologists (those who study the links between environment and lifestyle and disease) have observed that certain populations are largely free of heart disease while still enjoying relatively high amounts of fat. Early on, scientists were rather bewildered by these findings, since in those days the supposed problem was total fat, not specific fats. Greenland Eskimo consumed huge quantities of fat in their diet of fish and marine mammals, yet their language had no word for heart disease. But when Eskimo peoples moved to Denmark and took on westernized lifestyles, heart disease rates soared. People from Greece and other Mediterranean countries enjoyed olive oil, nuts, lots of fish and seafood, and some cheeses, but they had a very low rate of CHD. Genetically lucky people? No. When they moved from rural regions to the cities, they discovered fried fast foods, fatty meats, and dairy products, and they too developed the disease.

As time went on, scientists came to realize that consumption of saturated fats was actually as low as what American medical authorities were beginning to advocate, or even lower. Then the research became more specific, and the question was asked: Can such diets be adapted and adopted by people in the United States and elsewhere?

The resounding answer was definitely yes. Certainly we can all increase our intake of fruits, vegetables, and grains. Studies demonstrated that even small quantities of regularly consumed fish offered tremendous protection. Those following a modified version of the Mediterranean diet, which included a lot more monounsaturated fats in foods such as olives and nuts, instead of the saturated fats in full-fat dairy foods and meats, reaped the benefits of lowered blood pressure, less likelihood of forming blood clots, and lower levels of both total and LDL cholesterol. Yet their HDL counts remained high and their triglycerides stayed down.

A wonderful study putting a number of various dietary approaches under the microscope was undertaken at Penn State University. Renowned nutrition researcher Dr. Penny Kris-Etherton and her associates directly compared the effects of four different diets. First was the average American diet (AA), consisting of 34 percent total fat, 16 percent saturated fatty acids (SFAs), and 11 percent monounsaturated fats (MUFAs). The second diet was that advocated by the American Heart Association, which contained 25 percent total fat, 7 percent SFAs, and 12 percent MUFAs. That's called the Step II diet, for those with elevated cholesterol levels and perhaps a history of cardiac events. Dr. Kris-Etherton's third diet accentuated MUFAs. Total fat was 34 percent (just like the AA diet), but it replaced a lot of the saturated fats of meats and dairy with the MUFAs of olives and olive oil. A fourth diet was similar but used peanuts, peanut butter, and peanut oil.

Calories in all cases remained the same. Here's the bottom line: The MUFA diets lowered total cholesterol by 10 percent and LDL by 14 percent, about the same as the Step II diet. But triglycerides were 13 percent lower on the MUFA diet, compared with the AA diet, while the Step II diet raised triglycerides by 11 percent. MUFA diets did not lower HDL counts, while the Step II diet led to a 4 percent decrease. Not bad for a diet that's lots tastier!

But what about risk of heart disease? The Step II diet lowered CHD risk by 12 percent. That's good. But the MUFA diet with olive oil dropped CHD risk by 25 percent. And the diet with peanuts and peanut butter produced a 21 percent risk reduction.

Those results were published in the *American Journal of Clinical Nutrition* in December 1999. So there you are—the days of preferring a slice of bread or a serving of pasta over MUFA-rich foods are over. I now regularly bring a peanut butter and jelly sandwich on whole-grain bread with me to my weekend golf games. Ah, the victorious return of an all-American favorite!

Choosing the Best Fats and Oils

If any food product has survived the test of time, it's olive oil. Used healthfully for centuries, we now know that olive oil can lower cholesterol without adversely affecting levels of the protective HDL. Corn oil and others rich in polyunsaturated, rather than monounsaturated, fatty acids tend to lower both LDL and HDL cholesterol. And recent research has shown that olive oil as a regular part of the diet brings blood pressure down as well. Sunflower oil had no effects on blood pressure.

Regardless of quality or price, the fatty acid profile is the same for all olive oils. Enjoy extra-virgin olive oil on salads and whenever you want the full flavor. Ordinary olive oil is fine for sautéing. As for "lite" olive oil, it isn't light in either fat or calories. The term refers to the bland flavor and color. "Lite" olive oil is actually the cheapest and lowest quality, although it is sometimes sold at a premium price.

For those times when you want little or no flavor, your better choice would be canola oil, also extremely high in monounsaturated fatty acids. It works well for most kitchen purposes, including baking. You'll see it called for in many of my recipes at the back of the book. And because it has no adverse effects on my cholesterol level, I now use it in baking my oat bran muffins and cookies. They taste a whole lot better now!

Grapeseed oil attracted a lot of attention in the mid-1990s. Preliminary research done at the State University of New York in Syracuse indicated that it might be superior in actually raising HDL counts, rather than merely not lowering them as is the case for the monounsaturated-fat-rich olive and canola oils. But that research has never been replicated and confirmed. Interestingly, grapeseed oil is sold in the United States as a gourmet item in specialty stores. In Australia and elsewhere, it is as common (and inexpensive) as corn oil is here.

Now, all this should not make you feel that you should never use anything but olive or canola oils. If you have a preference for sunflower, soybean, or other oils, feel free to use them in good health. For a complete analysis of the fatty acid composition of cooking oils, see Table 2 (page 78).

Shopping for margarine is a little trickier. Stick margarines are made with hydrogenated oils to form the harder product. Hydrogenation brings with it increases in the amount of both saturated fat and trans fatty acids. The latter, covered in more detail in the coming pages, is actually worse than saturated fat, not only raising LDL cholesterol but lowering the good HDL type. Nasty stuff. Avoid it by using tub, spray, or squeeze-bottle margarines. And forget any nonsense that butter is better than margarine because it is more natural. Half of butter's fat is saturated. Stay away from it most of the time.

It's one thing to read the results of well-controlled laboratory studies, but what about in your own life and home, you might ask. Does using the right margarines and oils make a difference in real life? Australian researchers put that notion to the test, albeit with a rather captive audience.

They worked with members of the Australian National Antarctic Research Expedition during the winter of 1991. Those guys ate the food they were given—they couldn't exactly slip off to a restaurant or grocery store. During a 13-week trial, canola margarine and canola cooking oil were substituted for the usual dietary fats, which included butter, a stick margarine containing 28 percent saturated fat, and vegetable oil, Total cholesterol on average fell 7 percent and LDL went down to 10 percent. Conversely, another wintering group was given the usual fats and oils and they did not experience the cholesterol improvements. The Aussie investigators concluded that "a relatively simple change to the food supply has the potential to produce significant changes."

Avoiding the Bad Fats

Just because the monounsaturated fats help lower cholesterol counts doesn't mean that you should take a drink of olive oil to wash away the effects of a fast-food cheeseburger and fries. Ultimately it's a matter of replacing a lot of that saturated fat with the monounsaturated and polyunsaturated kinds.

I won't belabor the point or bore you with details of study after study, proving unequivocally that saturated fats raise total and LDL cholesterol levels dramatically. Suffice it to say that there have now been literally hundreds of papers published in the world's most prestigious journals that prove the point.

You want to cut your consumption of those saturated fats as much as possible. They are found in full-fat dairy products and fatty cuts of meat as well as in coconut and palm kernel; ironically, palm oil does *not* raise cholesterol levels as often as supposed. Fortunately, today you can easily substitute nonfat or low-fat versions of virtually all dairy products. There's even a nonfat half-and-half made by Land o' Lakes to use in coffee, cereal, or desserts. And with a little planning, you can have any cut of beef that has the fat content of a skinless chicken breast. (See "Listening to Your Inner Carnivore.")

We've talked about the good fats and the bad fats. Now let's talk about the ugly. That distinction belongs to a special, yet extremely commonplace, type of fat called trans fatty acids. This fat does not exist in nature. It is created when food manufacturers begin with an ordinary oil such as soybean or cottonseed oil and then hydrogenate it to turn the oil into a solid or semisolid state. This process chemically alters the fat, rearranging its molecules in what turns out to be a very deadly manner.

Over the past few years, the body of evidence showing the adverse effects of trans fatty acids has grown by leaps and bounds. We now know that these Frankenstein fats not only raise levels of total and LDL cholesterol but also lower HDL counts. This wreaks havoc with the cholesterol risk ratio and increases the danger of developing CHD.

Currently, trans fatty acids are not listed on the nutrition facts label of processed foods. The only way you know that they're there is by glancing at the ingredients list for the words "hydrogenated" or "partially hydrogenated" oils. Several consumer advocacy groups have lobbied the Food and Drug Administration to require specific listing of these fats. This will probably happen, but as yet there is no timetable.

In the meantime, it's best to avoid trans fatty acids as much as possible, since they are truly worse for your arteries than saturated fats—even worse than the tropical oils. Unfortunately, complete avoidance is very difficult since the trans fats are found in virtually all cookies, crackers, baked goods, desserts, and snacks. And virtually all fried fast foods in commercial outlets—French fries, chicken nuggets, fried chicken, and so on—are loaded with trans fats.

Have I personally eliminated 100 percent of trans fats from my own diet? No, but I have definitely cut back. Complete elimination would require more dedication and deprivation than even I am willing to endure. For example, I enjoy reduced-fat Triscuit crackers with herring as a snack or predinner appetizer. A serving (7 crackers) provides a nice healthy 4 grams of fiber. The total fat is listed as 3 grams; 0.5 gram of that is saturated and 1 gram as monounsaturated. What happened to the remaining 1.5 grams of fat? Those are the trans fats created by Triscuit's partially hydrogenated soybean oil.

Here's an easy way to determine your own trans fat intake. Read the labels of foods in the way I've shown in the Triscuit example.

Whatever fat is "missing" when you tally up the numbers of grams declared on the label should be considered trans fat.

In the old days, heart-healthy men and women had to keep track of the gram count of all fats. Today we've seen that this isn't really necessary. But we do want to limit the amount of saturated and trans fats in the diet. Consider them together as the "terrible twosome" when making food choices.

Putting It All Together

I guess one way to follow a heart-healthy Mediterranean diet would be to move to a Mediterranean island and eat like the locals. Not very practical? Well, how about building an igloo way up north and living on a diet of fish and marine mammals like seal and walrus? Not ready for that either? Nor am I. Actually, it's a lot easier than it might first appear to take full advantage of what we know about the good, the bad, and the ugly fats.

To put fats into their proper perspective, first consider the entire daily diet. Over the course of the day and throughout the week, you'll make food choices that will provide the nutrients you need within the limits of the total caloric intake to maintain a healthy weight.

Where will most of those calories and nutrients come from? The foundation of the modern, heart-healthy diet will be a large amount of fruits, vegetables, cereals, and grains. To that you will add two or perhaps three servings of nonfat and low-fat dairy foods, including milk, cheese, and yogurt. Next will be selections of protein-rich foods, including low-fat meats (beef, pork, and veal), poultry (white meat, no skin), and fish and seafood. Beans and legumes also count as protein foods and play a large role for those who choose vegetarianism.

Depending on your own caloric needs and limitations, you can enjoy the vast majority of fats and oils without any consideration of the fat grams you're consuming. I think that's pretty neat. Enjoy caesar salads with olive oil and a sprinkling of parmesan cheese. Sauté vegetables in canola oil. Don't even think about the fat in fish such as salmon, herring, sardines, mackerel, and so forth. In fact, choose the fattiest cuts of salmon you can find—they are the tastiest and actually the best for you! Don't bother with fat listings for cereals such as oatmeal and oat bran, unless the ingredients label indicates that hydrogenated oils have been added. Snack on nuts of all kinds. Enjoy a peanut butter sandwich as often as you wish. Try it with sliced bananas and a little honey for a change.

When it comes to sugar and honey, let your waistline be your guide. Sweets have virtually no nutrient value and add up in calories quickly, but they sure do taste good. Food is a blessing, a gift, a joy of life. Enjoy it in moderation.

And now we come to the only real limitations for a heart-healthy diet—saturated fats and trans fatty acids. Consider them together in determining your daily intake. The number of daily grams of saturated/trans fats depends on your total caloric needs. That, in turn, depends on a number of factors, including age, gender, body type, and daily physical activity.

As we age, we require fewer and fewer calories to maintain our bodies. Women, for the most part, do not burn as many calories as men, owing to a lower mass of lean muscle tissue. Only muscle, not fat, bone, or anything else, can burn calories. The higher the muscle mass, the greater the caloric allowance. A 200-pound big-boned athlete will burn far more calories than a sedentary man or woman of the same weight. And, obviously, the more physical activity and exercise a person gets, the more calories he or she can afford.

So let's take two examples—the same ones used on all nutrition facts labels on the foods you buy and use. For someone requiring 2000 calories a day, saturated/trans fat intake should be no more than 20 grams daily. On a 2500-calorie diet, that number rises to 25 grams. Those numbers are calculated as 10 percent of calories coming from saturated/trans fats.

The emphasis here must be on the phrase "no more than." The lower the saturated/trans fat intake, the better for your heart. As a 160-pound, fairly active male in my late fifties, my daily limit is about 15 grams. Many days it's lower.

Which brings us to the next topic. There is no little meter inside your body signaling that once you eat a certain number of grams of saturated/trans fat for the day, you start clogging your arteries. What really matters is not what you eat at any given meal, or on any given day, but, rather, what you eat on average week in and week out.

Let's say you've been really "good" all week. You've started your days with hot or cold cereals, fruit, juice, and skim milk most mornings. Lunches have included low-fat sandwiches, fruit, and salads or low-fat soups. You've had fish twice for dinner, and other days your evening meals have been healthfully chosen, with plenty of vegetables. So when the weekend comes along you might just want to splurge a little. The steak on the restaurant menu sounds really delicious. Go for it! Again, it's not the amount of trans fats you eat in one day but the average over a period of time.

With that in mind, I offer just one note of caution. It can be very easy to become lulled into complacency. That "once in a while" treat can become an all too regular thing. Today it's an anniversary, tomorrow a business lunch, the next day dinner at a friend's house where you don't want to "insult" the host by not eating everything offered. The key word is moderation.

I've been at this now since 1984, when I learned that I needed that second coronary bypass operation. Believe me when I say that after a while, perhaps two or three months, your improved diet will become a matter of habit. Trust me on this.

Now you may have noticed that I've hardly mentioned cholesterol in the diet. There is no question that large amounts of dietary cholesterol raise levels of cholesterol in the blood. Not as dramatically as saturated or trans fats, but very significantly. Happily, however, cholesterol is one of the easiest things to control.

First, only animal foods, both meats and dairy, contain cholesterol. There is absolutely none in any plant, fruit, vegetable, grain, cereal, or oil. As you begin to eat more plant-based foods and fewer and smaller servings of animal foods, you'll automatically cut back on dietary cholesterol without even thinking about it.

Second, lower-fat meats and dairy foods have smaller amounts of cholesterol per serving. Shellfish such as scallops and oysters have virtually no fat at all, and half the amount of cholesterol found in skinless chicken breast. And the ultra-low-fat beef I use and highly recommend has far less cholesterol than the leanest cuts of beef in the supermarket.

Third, and most important of all, you can actually block the absorption of cholesterol from the foods you eat so that it never enters the bloodstream. It's a matter of counteracting the cholesterol, an animal sterol, with phytosterol, a plant sterol. The body can't tell the difference between the two, and thus taking a phytosterol supplement with meals can very effectively keep the cholesterol in your food from getting into your bloodstream.

THE FAT PRIMER

All fats and oils are composed of fatty acids, which are chains of carbon atoms of varying lengths and hydrogen atoms. The more hydrogen atoms in the fatty acid molecule, the more saturated it is said to be.

No fat or oil is composed exclusively of just one type of fatty acid. Rather, fats and oils are a mix of fatty acids that are saturated (completely filled with hydrogen atoms), polyunsaturated (some carbon atoms without hydrogen atoms), and monounsaturated (one carbon atom with a hydrogen bond).

Saturated fats tend to be solid or semisolid at room temperature. Foods and edible oils containing a large percentage of saturated fatty acids include butter, animal fat, and the tropical oils (palm, palm kernel, and coconut). Ironically, however, the particular type of saturated fat in palm oil, palmitic acid, does not raise cholesterol levels. The villains are lauric and myristic acids, found in butter, other animal fats, and both coconut and palm kernel oils. The foods rich in saturated fats have been clinically proven to raise levels of cholesterol in the bloodstream.

Polyunsaturated fats are liquid at room temperature and tend to remain in a liquid state even at cooler temperatures. Foods and edible oils containing a large percentage of polyunsaturated fatty acids include corn oil, sunflower oil, soybean oil, safflower oil, and fish oils. The latter have a special type of polyunsaturated fatty acids termed omega-3. Flaxseed is a plant source of omega-3 fat.

Monounsaturated fats are thicker liquids or semisolid at room or cooler temperatures. Foods and edible oils containing a large percentage of monounsaturated fatty acids include olives, various kinds of nuts, avocados, olive oil, and canola oil.

Trans fatty acids do not exist in nature. They are formed when oils are hydrogenated by manufacturers for use in margarines, shortenings, baked goods of all sorts, a variety of processed foods, and commercially prepared fired foods such as those in fast-food outlets. Foods containing trans fatty acids pose the danger of raising cholesterol levels in the bloodstream while at the same time lowering levels of protective HDL.

Don't Be Fooled by "Thin" Oil

Some manufacturers called them "zero-fat oils." Others claim they will help you lose weight. They are all oils made with primarily medium-chain triglycerides (MCTs), and not only do they not work as claimed, they may actually be bad for you.

These oils were originally designed for hospitalized patients fed through a tube and for those with rare malabsorption syndromes. Ironically, then, they are meant for those who require *more* calories, not fewer. MCTs supply 8.3 calories per gram, just slightly less than ordinary oils. The real difference is that they are metabolized more like carbohydrates and are absorbed directly into the liver.

It is true that MCTs do not raise cholesterol levels. But that is also true for all other cooking oils.

MCT oils are hideously expensive. But the trouble doesn't stop there. They do not supply essential fatty acids needed by the body. MCTs can lead to gastrointestinal upset. And they can be a particular problem for those with liver troubles. Forget them.

Table 2. **Comparison of Dietary Fats and Oils**

	Saturated Fatty Acids (% of total)*	Monounsaturated Fatty Acids (% of total)*	Polyunsaturated Fatty Acids (% of total)*
Canola oil	6	62	32
Grapeseed oil	8	16	72
Walnut oil	9	23	64
Safflower oil	10	13	77
Sunflower oil	11	20	69
Corn oil	13	25	62
Olive oil	14	77	9
Soybean oil	15	24	61
Peanut oil	18	49	33
Margarine (tub)	18	47	31
Cottonseed oil	27	19	54
Tuna fat	27	26	21
Chicken fat	30	45	11
Margarine (stick)	31	47	22
Shortening (can)	31	51	14
Lard	40	45	11
Mutton fat	47	41	8
Palm oil	49	37	9
Beef fat	50	42	4
Butterfat	62	29	4
Palm kernel oil	81	11	2
Coconut oil	86	6	2

* Percentages are averaged and thus may not total exactly 100 percent.

A NUTTY APPROACH TO HEART HEALTH

The news coming out of Loma Linda University in the early 1990s seemed more than a little strange to those of us who had been preaching the low-fat gospel for years. Dr. Gary Fraser reported that those who regularly snacked on nuts, about a handful a day, had a significantly lower risk of CHD than those who avoided nuts.

How could that be? Nuts of all kinds are notoriously high in fat. One ounce packs from 13 to 19 grams of fat. Bear in mind that an ounce is the equivalent of 28 grams. So about half of the weight—and calories—of nuts comes from fat.

Of course, most of that fat is polyunsaturated and monounsaturated, so it was assumed that those nut lovers were eating these snacks instead of other foods that contain more saturated fats. The advice continued to be to keep nut munching down to a once-in-a-while moderate intake because we were still concerned about the potential dangers of the day's total fat consumption.

But the research data kept coming in. Peanuts actually had a cholesterol-lowering effect. So did walnuts. Then almonds. And even macadamia nuts. Those who enjoyed nuts frequently had less CHD risk. Moreover, it wasn't just a matter of replacement of saturated fats, since the total fat intake was actually higher than authorities normally advise.

Researchers at the University of Hawaii found that a nut-filled diet providing 37 percent of calories from fat did as good a job of lowering cholesterol as a 30 percent fat diet. Their subjects munched on macadamias.

Doctors in Barcelona, Spain, were pleased to find that walnuts were good for their patients. They compared diets that contained a lot of nuts—8 to 11 walnuts daily—to one without nuts that contained the same amount of fat. The control diet had a lot of olives and olive oil, typical of the Mediterranean pattern. Both diets brought down total and LDL cholesterol, but nuts did a better job. LDL counts fell by 5.6 percent on the Mediterranean diet and by 11.2 percent on the walnut-inclusive diet.

Then in July 2001, researchers from the University of California at Davis published that walnuts, when added to both regular and low-fat diets, significantly lowered total as well as LDL cholesterol. The doctors feel that the fat balance in walnuts actually has a cholesterol-lowering effect, working by way of a mechanism much different from simply replacing saturated fats from other foods.

Finally, the most complete and well-designed research project of all delivered the conclusion that nuts can and should be part of a heart-healthy diet. That study was undertaken by Dr. Penny Kris-Etherton at Penn State. Essentially, those enjoying a high-fat diet rich in peanuts and peanut oil did better than those on a lower-fat diet, both in terms of cholesterol control and reduction of CHD risk.

Why are nuts so good for us? Well, of course the fat is mainly unsaturated. But there's apparently more to it than that. Alpha-linoleic acid, one of the fatty acid components that make up the total fat in nuts, reduces the tendency to form blood clots and regulates healthy heartbeat rhythms. Nuts are also rich in the amino acid arginine, necessary for the body's production of a chemical called nitric oxide that keeps the lining of arteries healthy, elastic, and able to dilate, allowing for greater blood flow when needed. As time goes on, we'll probably learn even more reasons to adopt this nutty approach to heart health.

Just a small note of caution that will come as no real surprise. As you can see in Table 3, nuts are quite high in calories. Don't get carried away.

As to the best nut, it's entirely a matter of taste. Especially during the winter holidays, I enjoy having a bowl of mixed nuts—walnuts, almonds, hazelnuts—on the table in the family room. It's fun to crack the nuts and munch while entertaining or watching TV. And the effort of cracking and picking the nuts tends to limit the total amount eaten!

Table 3. **Fat and Calorie Composition of Nuts**

Nuts and Nut Butters*	Calories	Fat (grams)
Almonds	175	14.5
Brazil	186	18.8
Cashew	163	13.0
Filbert/hazelnut	188	18.8
Peanuts	164	13.9
Pecans	187	18.0
Almond butter	190	18.0
Cashew butter	190	15.0
Peanut butter	188	16.0

* Amounts are as follows: nuts, 1 ounce, dry roasted (oil adds 1 gram per ounce); nut butters, 2 tablespoons

LISTENING TO YOUR INNER CARNIVORE

Despite the loud clamor of a vocal minority, humans were not meant to be herbivores (vegetarians). We have teeth quite capable of ripping meat off the bone, some very specialized enzymes to digest the meat, and an intestinal tract that gets the nutrients out into the bloodstream for use.

Clearly, however, we're not meant to be exclusively carnivorous. We couldn't live on meat alone. Conversely, a strictly vegetarian (vegan) diet that contains no meat or dairy is likely to be deficient in iron, calcium, and vitamin B_{12}. Like a raccoon or bear, we are designed to be omnivores, eating from both the plant and the animal kingdoms.

Anthropologists digging into our ancestral past have uncovered vast piles of oyster and clam shells and mounds of bones from which meat was hacked or chewed, either raw or, later in our prehistory, cooked. Many scientists believe that cooked meats, with their denser supply of nutrients, gave early humans the time that would otherwise have been spent gathering and chewing plants to develop our abilities as tool makers, artisans, and explorers.

Meats eaten at the dawn of our existence were indeed healthy sources of nutrition. Fish and shellfish are low in fat yet high in protein and other nutrients. The same holds for wild game such as birds, antelope, buffalo, rabbits, squirrels, and pigs. The trouble began when humans domesticated those animals and fattened them up, penned them in, and fed them grains. A wild mallard duck is very low in fat, while domestic duckling drips with it. Then there's prime beef and fattened pork. Early farmers, and later ranchers, found meat tasted better that way, and they didn't know much about nutrition. Today many meats are major sources of saturated fat and cholesterol.

So it's no surprise that dieticians, nutritionists, and physicians respond to a patient's high cholesterol count by advising them to cut back on meat—or even eliminate it altogether. Sadly, they're throwing the baby out with the bath water, apparently not realizing there are wonderful ways to get rid of the fat and keep the taste and nutrition of meat.

Researchers in Chicago compared the effects of a diet that included lean cuts of meat with a vegetarian diet. Good news! Total and LDL cholesterol fell equally well. In fact, meat eaters fared better, since their HDL levels did not go down and their triglycerides did not go up. This was not the case for the high-carbohydrate vegetarian dieters.

Look at the dietary guidelines issued by the American Heart Association, the American Dietetic Association, and practically every other health organization other than those with a hidden animal rights agenda. They all call for a diet that includes lean meat, poultry, and seafood. In fact, the 2000 AHA guidelines specifically recommend at least two fatty fish meals weekly. The bottom line is this: there is no good scientific reason not to enjoy all sorts of meat as part of a heart-healthy lifestyle.

If you happen to be a hunter, or know one who might bring wild game to your kitchen, terrific. Virtually all game is extremely low in fat and cholesterol. And if you enjoy wild game but don't have a hunter handy, you can do your own hunting with a credit card and a telephone or a computer. (Wild game suppliers are listed on page 84.)

But most of us seek our meat in the supermarket. Statistics from the U.S. Department of Agriculture show that more than half of all red meat consumed in this country is in the form of ground beef. So let's start there.

Standard ground beef, by USDA standards, is 30 percent fat. Lean ground beef brings that number down to 22 percent. Very lean means 15 percent. And many supermarkets are now offering 90 percent lean (10 percent fat) and even 93 percent lean (7 percent fat) for health-conscious customers.

You can get your ground beef even leaner. Just select a chunk of round steak, London broil, or top sirloin from the meat section. Then ask the butcher to first trim off the visible fat and then grind it. Bingo. You're down to a mere 5 percent fat. You can do the same with a chunk of pork loin, to make sausage or meatloaf or Swedish meatballs.

Think about all the uses you have weekly for ground beef—spaghetti sauce, chili, hamburgers, tacos and other Mexican dishes. You can see tremendous fat-lowering potential by making this one simple change. I like to buy a large amount, say 10 pounds or so, when lean cuts are on sale, then divide the ground beef into 1-pound packages for the freezer.

A bit too dry, you might wonder? No problem. With today's revised views of cooking oils, it's easy to add back some of the fat by sautéing the ground beef with healthier canola or olive oil. Or add some oil to the meatloaf or hamburger mixture.

Want a steak, either from the supermarket or at a restaurant? Choose a cut with the word *loin* or *round* in the name such as sirloin, tenderloin, or top sirloin. Those are the lowest in fat.

Veal is another good choice. Choose a well-trimmed veal chop, stew meat, cutlets, and medallions.

When it comes to pork, eat "high on the hog." That expression dates back to a time when the more expensive cuts came from the upper portion of the animal and cheaper cuts were those from the lower portion. While those lower cuts, including bacon, are high in fat, the upper cuts—loin, ham, and tenderloin—are actually quite low. Tenderloin comes in at about 4 percent fat, trimmed and loin cuts are 5 to 6 percent; ham varies quite a lot, so be sure to read the label.

Very Special Beef

Sometimes nature plays tricks with animals' genes, creating new species or breeds. That's the case with two types of beef cattle—Belgian Blue from Belgium and France and Piedmontese from Italy. Both have a chromosomal abnormality (abnormal in a good way) that results in a condition known as double muscling. These animals are the hulking "linebackers" of the cattle world—very high in muscle and protein, very low in fat. In fact, there's no more fat than in skinless chicken breast. And that holds true for all the cuts, not just the round and loin. So you can enjoy rib-eye steaks, New York strips, brisket, short ribs, you name it.

But what about taste and tenderness? Other types of low-fat beef are simply raised on grass rather than grain to get the fat content down. And some ranchers crossbreed with animals lower in fat such as Charólais and Simenthal. Unfortunately, such beef tends to be tough and tasteless.

The Belgian Blue and Piedmontese cattle, on the other hand, are naturally lean yet tender. That's because the individual muscle fibers, while larger in number, are shorter. Laboratory tests have shown tenderness, measured in what's called "shear force," is just short of prime beef, the fattiest of them all. Yet this meat is extremely low in fat. And it tastes marvelous.

Another remarkable quality is that in the ground beef hamburgers, virtually all the fat, not just some, drips off during cooking. So you can throw a 13 percent fat hamburger patty on the grill or under the broiler and it comes out delicious and practically free of fat.

As time goes on, it is expected that this wonderful beef will be in many supermarkets. Already some upscale restaurants have begun to feature it on their menus. But for now the best way to get either type is by mail order over the phone. Prices are not at all exorbitant.

Expect to pay what you would in a good butcher shop, plus the shipping costs.

Because this beef is extremely low in fat, it cooks much faster than ordinary meat. That's because fat acts as an insulator and slows the cooking process. Broil or grill this meat in about half the time you would expect.

This beef is best enjoyed rare or medium rare to be at its juiciest and tastiest. You'll have better results, as is true with all beef, cooking up thicker steaks. When placing an order, rather than asking for two 8-ounce steaks, which will be on the thin side, get one 16-ounce slab that you can cut in half after cooking.

As an added bonus, Belgian Blue and Piedmontese cattle are raised without the use of hormones and antibiotics. You have here the healthiest beef you can buy. Imagine being able to enjoy all your favorite beef cuts and recipes, from short ribs to roasts to brisket—you name it!

For Piedmontese beef, phone in orders toll-free at 877-332-4222 or visit their Web site at www.olympianfoods.com. Order Belgian Blue beef at 877-425-8363. Which is better? I'd suggest a taste test. Get a few different cuts of both types of beef and see which you prefer. In my opinion, both are delicious and I enjoy this beef literally every week.

For wild and exotic game meats, including buffalo, ostrich, elk, and so forth, try American Bison Meat at 800-789-3044. Another very excellent source of wild game meats of all sorts from literally all over the world is Nicky USA Inc. Contact them at 503-234-GAME in Oregon, or 800-469-4162. Even if you're just curious, you'll enjoy their Web site. Log on to www.nickyusawildgame.com to check out everything from alligator to kangaroo to turtle. This one will definately bring out the Paleolithic carnivore in you!

Heart Health Your Wish? Put Fish on Your Dish!

I find it astounding that anyone who regularly reads the scientific and medical literature could still recommend a vegetarian diet free of fish and seafood. For years, the idea of fish being "heart food" came from observations of people who ate or didn't eat fish. Now the evidence is so clear that the AHA recommends having fatty fish twice a week.

First, of course, we heard about the Eskimos and how they almost never developed heart disease even though they ate large amounts of fat in the form or fish and marine animals. Then a long-term study of workers at the Western Electric Company in Chicago hinted that fish lovers enjoyed protection against CHD. The risk of fatal heart attack was slashed by a third just from this one lifestyle factor. A similar investigation that examined the habits of tens of thousands of male physicians revealed that those who ate fish at least once a week had half the risk of sudden cardiac death.

The list of research studies goes on and on, all with favorable results. We know now that the major fish oils, eicosapentanoic acid (EPA) and docosahexanoic acid (DHA), work in a number of wonderful ways. These omega-3 fatty acids reduce the formation of blood clots and raise levels of the protective HDL cholesterol while dramatically lowering triglycerides. In addition they prevent potentially fatal heart rhythm disturbances. (See Table 4 for omega-3 levels of various fish.)

In my book in 1987, I heartily encouraged eating fish as often as possible, saying the fattier the fish the better since that fat did not count. But I drew the line at fish oil supplements. There just wasn't enough evidence that the isolated oils in pills would do the job of real, naturally occurring omega-3 fatty acids. Besides, there might be other factors in fish that contribute to the protection. And we didn't know much about potential adverse reactions.

That was then and this is now. While I still urge you to eat and enjoy fish, including salmon, herring, mackerel, bluefish, sardines, and other fatty varieties, those who simply do not like fish can turn to pills. Research within the past few years has shown that they provide similar benefits. Look for supplements that provide about 4 grams of EPA and DHA daily. One study showed that this amount could potentially reduce the risk of CHD by 27 percent in postmenopausal women. Another demonstrated that the supplements improved the arteries' ability to dilate, providing greater blood flow. Still another found that EPA and DHA lowered triglyceride levels, changed the molecular structure of cholesterol molecules in the bloodstream to a less dangerous size and density, and reduced both glucose and insulin in men with mild cases of increased amounts of fats in their blood. Other research indicates that supplements reduce symptoms of arthritis.

One of the early concerns, that of potentially raising total and LDL levels, has been dismissed. The major downside to oil capsules is that the large doses needed to get favorable results often lead to fishy breath and the unpleasant experience of oil being regurgitated into the mouth. And fish oil doesn't taste very good at all. For myself, I'll stick with fish, which I truly enjoy.

Other Treats from the Sea

In the early days of dietary recommendations to prevent CHD, shellfish were on the no-no list. Oysters, clams, scallops, and the like were said to be extremely high in cholesterol. It turns out that was an error. Devices used to measure cholesterol in animal tissue were erroneously counting plant sterols eaten by the shellfish as cholesterol, giving wrong information. Actually those shellfish are extremely *low* in cholesterol and virtually devoid of fat (see Table 5).

Table 4. **Omega-3 Fatty-Acid Content**

	Amount*
Sardines (Norway)	5.1
Sockeye salmon	2.7
Mackerel (Atlantic)	2.5
King Salmon	1.9
Herring	1.7
Lake trout	1.4
Albacore tuna	1.3
Halibut	1.3
Bluefish	1.2
Mackerel (Pacific)	1.1
Striped Bass	0.8
Yellowfin tuna	0.6
Pollock	0.5
Brook trout	0.4
Yellow perch	0.3
Catfish	0.2

Table 5. **Calorie, Fat, and Cholesterol Content of Shellfish***

	Calories	Fat	Cholesterol
Abalone	195	0.7 g	85 mg
Clams	74	1.0 g	34 mg
Crayfish	90	1.1 g	139 mg
Mussels	86	2.2 g	28 mg
Oysters	69	2.5 g	55 mg
Scallops	88	0.8 g	33 mg
Alaska crab	84	0.6 g	42 mg
Maine lobster	90	0.9 g	95 mg
Rock lobster (spiny)	112	1.5 g	70 mg
Shrimp	106	1.7 g	152 mg

* Based on servings of 3.5 ounces (100 grams), raw.

The same holds true for crab and lobster. However, shrimp are on the high side, as are abalone and squid (calamari). Fortunately, there is a very convenient way to block the absorption of the cholesterol in such foods from ever entering the bloodstream, as described on page 117.

SOY FOODS AND THE HEART

Vegetarians have long touted the benefits of soy, citing all sorts of health advantages. Until recently, however, anyone who talked about tofu or tempeh was thought to be a health nut. Now we're seeing all sorts of foods and supplements in mainstream supermarkets, fueled by positive media reporting on soy.

In 1999, the Food and Drug Administration approved use of a health claim for foods containing soy protein. Food products with a minimum of 6.25 grams of soy protein per serving are now allowed to feature one of two wordings on labels:

> "25 grams of soy protein a day, as part of a diet low in saturated fat and cholesterol, may reduce the risk of heart disease. A serving of _____ supplies _____ grams of soy protein."

or

> "Diets low in saturated fat and cholesterol that include 25 grams of soy protein a day may reduce the risk of heart disease. One serving of _____ provides _____ grams of soy protein."

In terms of nutrition, soy protein compares favorably with milk, meat, or eggs. In addition to tofu, tempeh, and miso, isolated soy protein is now commonly found in soy milk, soy nuts, soy cheeses, nutrition bars, and shake mixes. But how much can soy actually help your heart? The answer is a bit more complicated than typical newspaper articles reveal.

Yes, quite a few research studies have shown that soy can reduce cholesterol levels and the risk of CHD development. In 1995 Dr. James Anderson of the University of Kentucky pooled the data from 38 separate soy studies. Those getting an average of 47 grams of soy protein per day saw a decrease in total cholesterol of about 9 percent, and LDL levels fell by almost 13 percent. HDL rose slightly, and triglycerides came down between 10 and 11 percent. Improvements were most dramatic in those whose cholesterol measurements were relatively high to begin with.

So how much soy protein is enough to get some benefit? Asians average about 20 grams a day. That's a bit less than an ounce, which equals 28 grams. So 47 grams would double that intake. Bear in mind, also, that we're talking about the soy protein in foods, not the total weight of soy-based foods and beverages.

Lesser amounts do tilt the cholesterol balance in a positive direction, but not dramatically so. One study saw a drop in total and LDL cholesterol with 25 grams daily, but that was only in those with very high starting numbers. A report in 2000 concluded that 20 grams daily yielded a 2.6 percent reduction on average.

In all cases, we're talking about replacing animal proteins in foods such as meat, fish, poultry, and dairy with soy protein. It's not a matter of adding soy protein to an animal protein–based diet. So it's a question of whether you want to drink soy milk instead of regular milk and eat tofu rather than a chicken breast or beef burger. Moreover, do you want to make those replacements on a regular, daily basis? Just once in a while won't make a difference.

With those thoughts in mind, forget about swallowing soy supplements. You're just wasting your money. There's no proof that the isoflavones such as genestein in supplements can do the job of whole soy foods or foods to which soy protein has been added.

And contrary to popular opinion, soy does have a dark side. The isoflavone genestein is a plant estrogen. In fact, some women rely on soy as an alternative to hormone replacement therapy at menopause. That can be a good thing. But some cancers, including breast and prostate, are sensitive to estrogens of all sorts, including those from plant sources. Genistein could actually contribute to the development of those cancers.

Second, soy protein has been shown to increase levels of the really nasty variant of LDL called Lp(a), an independent risk factor for CHD. That was the finding of a Danish research team in 1999. I must say, however, that participants consumed large amounts of soy protein, about 150 grams daily, mixed into a liquid diet. When the soy protein was replaced by milk protein (casein), Lp(a) counts fell. But 150 grams of any one form of protein is excessively high. Moreover, to the best of my knowledge, that was the only study published showing the negative effects of soy on Lp(a).

It's quite possible that vegetarians who eat soy foods on a regular basis can reap some CHD protection. Eating soy foods now and then almost certainly won't make an impact on cholesterol levels or CHD risk. However, soy foods typically have far less fat in general, and less saturated fat in particular, than the animal foods they would replace, so that's good. The final word on soy? So-so.

GARLIC: WILL A CLOVE A DAY
KEEP THE DOCTOR AWAY?

There's always a good supply of garlic cloves in my kitchen, and I've never seen any vampires in my house, so maybe that herb keeps the bloodsuckers at bay. But it appears less likely that the "stinking rose" has much, if any, CHD protection.

Folk medicine touts garlic as a cure for practically anything that ails you. Scientists have been skeptical but some preliminary studies were promising. In 1993 doctors at the New York Medical College published their meta-analysis of garlic research, pooling data from a number of studies. They concluded that the equivalent of one-half to one clove of garlic daily resulted, on average, in a 9 percent reduction in total cholesterol. As an added benefit, garlic appeared to prevent excessive blood clotting and control high blood pressure as well.

That same year, Russian scientists gave glowing reports on how garlic limited uptake of LDL cholesterol. They grew artery-clogging atherosclerotic cells in laboratory dishes and found that garlic inhibited the growth of those artery-clogging cells. Their work was done with garlic powder, and human, or even animal, studies have not been done to confirm these in vitro ("in glass") experiments.

In 1995 German investigators announced that subjects' total cholesterol dropped by 8 to 12 percent after they took 600 to 900 mg of garlic as tablets. And the German Commission E, a nonprofit watchdog group that studies and reports on various herbal remedies, published a report that garlic was effective for cholesterol control.

That was all good news, but those studies didn't control for weight or fat consumption by participants. No long-term investigations had determined whether garlic's effects last for longer than three months. And no dosage studies were available to answer the inevitable question: if a little is good, is more better?

Unfortunately, garlic has not held up as well in recent studies. German researchers published a paper in 1998 saying that commercial garlic oil preparations had no influence on cholesterol or triglycerides. They concluded that "garlic therapy for treatment of hypercholesterolemia cannot be recommended on the basis of this study." And Commission E no longer advocates garlic for heart disease prevention or cholesterol control.

The vast majority of studies have shown no benefit from garlic in lowering blood pressure. Even in positive reports, improvements have been tiny.

Even research commissioned and paid for by garlic supplement companies have not been able to show cholesterol-lowering capabilities.

The biggest disappointment came when the Agency for Healthcare Research and Quality reported that garlic did not lower cholesterol on a long-term basis. While numbers fell during the first few months of usage, they crept back up by the end of a year. The report, done through the National Center for Complementary and Alternative Medicine, a component of the National Institutes of Health, also found no evidence that garlic has a beneficial effect on blood pressure or diabetes. Effects on blood clotting are sketchy.

Most studies have focused on supplements. Research involving actual garlic cloves might provide positive results. Perhaps the beneficial compounds in fresh garlic, or even powder, is lost when garlic is processed into tablets.

Some reputable scientific researchers still believe in garlic's value. Dr. Varro Tyler, an herbal expert at Purdue University, says there is no question that garlic inhibits blood clotting. He says it is as potent a blood thinner as aspirin.

We have not heard the last about garlic. But regardless of advertising claims by celebrities such as Larry King, it doesn't make much sense to spend your money on garlic supplements.

If anything, you may want to include garlic frequently in your diet. Certainly there could be no adverse effects, other than perhaps bad breath, and there are hundreds of delicious ways to add garlic to your diet. One of my favorites is to roast a whole head of garlic and squeeze the softened cloves onto bread for a wonderful spread at dinner. No fat, tons of flavor.

To try it, snip the tips off of a head of garlic and remove the papery layers. Brush lightly with olive oil and wrap the head in aluminum foil. (You can also find little pottery containers for the express purpose of roasting garlic heads.) Bake one hour at 350° Fahrenheit. Allow to cool a bit and then squeeze the pungent, semiliquid garlic onto the bread. Taste it once and I guarantee this delicacy will become a regular part of your diet.

You can also enhance practically any recipe calling for sautéed onions by adding a few cloves of minced garlic. Easy. Place the cloves on a cutting board, give them a whack with the flat side of a large knife or put the cloves under the knife and smack it with your hand to crack the husk so it's simple to peel off. Then either crush the cloves with the same knife or mince.

There's a saying in garlic-loving cultures that you can have too little garlic, or enough garlic, but never too much garlic in your food.

Will it help your heart? Maybe. Will it put a smile on your face? Absolutely!

LIFTING A GLASS TO HEART HEALTH

Throughout history, physicians have prescribed alcohol for its health benefits. Sumerian doctors suggested beer, Egyptian practitioners extolled the virtues of beer and wine, and Greek healers used herb-infused wine as medicine. Today we have the scientific proof that drinking in moderation is actually good for most people.

In most cases, one can find research studies to back up one side of an issue and other reports in defense of the opposite. As time goes on in the research process, more evidence piles up on one side than on the other and we come to a conclusion. Rarely do investigators come to the same conclusion in study after study, with little or no equivocation. But that's the situation with alcohol and heart health.

Data have come in from all over the world. Studies have focused on both men and women, various age groups, and people of many ethnic groups. The conclusion remains the same: those who drink moderately live longer and have less risk of developing heart disease than those who abstain from alcohol. Published papers now total in the many hundreds.

Still, some naysayers had their doubts. Perhaps the teetotalers previously drank excessively and had undermined their health, thus explaining their higher levels of risk. In response, later studies excluded all but those who had excluded alcohol for their entire lives. The conclusions remained the same: alcohol confers protection against CHD, and drinkers live longer than nondrinkers.

Some authorities feel the benefits of alcohol are so compelling that doctors should suggest it to their patients. Others fear the significant risks associated with abuse and alcoholism. So let's put the risks and benefits into proper perspective.

Alcohol and Your Heart

The first solid evidence of alcohol's protective benefits for the heart came from work done by Dr. Arthur Klatsky at Kaiser Permanente in California. In 1974 he found that abstainers suffered more heart attacks than drinkers. Three years later the Honolulu Heart Program demonstrated that those who never drank alcohol had twice the risk of heart disease as those who drank in moderation.

Later, two long-term Harvard investigations proved the benefits of alcohol for both men and women. In one, physicians who drank alcoholic beverages had fewer cardiac events, including heart attacks and bypass surgeries. Their risk was cut by about 30 percent. In the other, women in the Nurses' Health Study who drank in moderation received protection from heart disease.

The key word is moderation. Statistically speaking, average risk is rated as 1.0. During the 12 years of the Nurses' Health Study, women consuming 1 to 3 drinks weekly had a death risk of 0.83 when compared with nondrinkers. Women drinking more than 3 but fewer than 18 drinks a week had a 0.88 risk of death. But those consuming above 18 increased their risk to 1.19.

Moderate drinking is defined as having no more than two drinks per day. One drink is 1.5 ounces of hard liquor such as scotch or gin, a 12-ounce can or bottle of beer, or a 5-ounce glass of wine.

Moderate drinking for women means no more than one drink daily. Risk of breast cancer goes up with higher alcohol intakes and women have less of the specific enzyme that metabolizes alcohol.

Alcohol consumption and health can be described as a J-shaped curve. Enjoy one or two drinks daily and one's all-cause mortality drops, especially risk of cardiovascular disease. Drink three or more alcoholic beverages a day and the mortality rate rises. Although protection against heart disease remains the same, other causes of death increase.

Nor can one "save up" his or her drinks for a binge one or two nights a week. Drinking several alcoholic beverages in one day raises blood pressure, damages the heart's muscular walls, injures the liver, raises triglycerides, and can lead to injuries.

Alcohol confers its protection on the heart in a number of ways. First and foremost, the alcohol itself, whether from beer, wine, or spirits, raises levels of the protective HDL cholesterol. Within the limits of moderation, the more one drinks, the greater the HDL increase.

Next, alcohol interferes with formation of blood clots that can lead to a heart attack. When blood platelets are particularly sticky, they tend to form clots more readily. Alcohol makes those platelets less sticky. Second, a substance in blood called fibrinogen facilitates clotting; alcohol breaks down that fibrinogen, reducing levels in the blood and thus preventing excessive clotting. Third, a natural clot buster, tissue plasminogen activator (tPA), increases in the blood of drinkers. Interestingly, doctors inject doses of tPA to dissolve clots in patients having a heart attack, thus reestablishing blood flow.

Another method of protection centers on alcohol's ability to suppress the development of muscle cells in the lining of the arteries.

Excessive growth of those cells leads to narrowing of the arteries. And scientists currently believe that much of that cell growth happens after meals. But when alcohol accompanies the meal, development of cells drops by 20 percent, according to Swiss researchers in 1998. Alcoholic beverages of any kind affect the cellular inhibition.

Beer and wine also provide an antioxidant potential not present in spirits. Oxidized LDL cholesterol is most dangerous to the arteries. Experiments have shown that when LDL oxidation is blocked by antioxidants of one sort or another, less plaque forms in the arteries. Beer and red and white wine contain a number of potent antioxidants called flavonoids and phenols.

Only red wine contains resveratrol, an antioxidant compound formed when grape skins are left on during the fermentation period to give wine its red color. Some believe that resveratrol is responsible for the "French paradox"—the low levels of heart disease among the French despite a diet that includes butter, cream, cheeses, and paté.

Actually, the only real controversy regarding alcohol and heart health centers on which type of alcoholic beverage is best. Advocates ardently defend their own preference. Good, solid evidence backs everyone's position. Not surprisingly, much of the research showing the benefits of red wine comes from regions where that beverage is made and consumed. The same holds true for beer.

In his continuing research at Kaiser Permanente, Dr. Klatsky compared drinkers of red and white wines and found no difference in health benefits. Both groups had the edge over those who didn't drink at all. He notes, however, that wine drinkers tend to be more educated and affluent than those who choose other beverages and that such individuals are typically more health-conscious in general, smoking less and exercising more. Thus the lifestyles of wine drinkers may be more responsible for their better health than their drink preferences.

When it comes to antioxidants, however, no wine or beer can compare with fruits and vegetables. You can get as much or more of the protective resveratrol in red grape juice as you can from red wine. And it's a lot safer to quaff grape juice in the morning or afternoon than the wine. Significantly, the French consume many more fruits and vegetables than do Americans. But it's a lot more attention-getting to focus on wine.

Ultimately, the major benefits of regular, moderate alcohol consumption come from the alcohol itself and its ability to raise HDL counts and reduce blood clotting. So it's up to you to choose which you prefer. Personally, I like a bottle of beer with spicy Mexican, Chinese, or Indian foods. There's nothing like a good red wine with a juicy steak or Italian dishes. A simple piece of fish calls for a glass of white wine. And sometimes I prefer to linger over a cocktail or a scotch on the rocks as I chat with my wife before dinner about the events of the day. Variety is the spice of life. And a variety of alcoholic beverages can extend life.

Should Everyone Drink Alcohol?

Absolutely not. I've already mentioned women's added risk of breast cancer and you need to consider your family history. Anyone who, in the past, has had problems with excessive alcohol use will probably find it easier and healthier to stay away from it entirely. Doctors typically forbid or strictly limit alcohol for patients with seriously elevated blood pressure, and liquor can aggravate existing problems such as gout.

Headlines proclaim the possible role of red wine in the French paradox. But we seldom hear the fact that France has one of the world's highest rates of cirrhosis of the liver.

Alcohol not only contributes calories to the diet but also reduces inhibitions that would otherwise limit consumption of high-calorie, high-fat appetizers during cocktail hours, selection of a fatty entrée one would otherwise pass up, or the decision to indulge in a rich dessert.

It goes without saying that drinking and driving don't mix. The same goes for drinking while doing anything that calls for strict attention and motor skills.

Data in the March 10, 2001, issue of *The Lancet* revealed that heavy drinking raises levels of CRP, the protein linked with CHD. The effect was seen with three daily drinks or more.

Recent research gives the green light to those who were previously forbidden to drink. Contrary to general medical assumption, moderate alcohol consumption apparently does not harm, and may protect, patients with heart failure. In a study by Cooper et al. published by the *American College of Cardiology* in May 2000, those who consumed 1 to 14 drinks per week had a 15 percent reduction in the rate of all-cause mortality and a 45 percent difference in death due to heart attack.

Doctors have traditionally instructed patients with diabetes not to drink. But 1999 research provides the okay for those with Type 2 (mature onset) diabetes to indulge moderately. Diabetic drinkers had a significantly lower rate of death from heart attack than nondrinkers. Protection increased as subjects consumed alcohol more frequently, with those having a drink daily being at the least risk.

Conversely, light to moderate drinking does *not* have the same cardiovascular benefits in men with established coronary heart disease as it does in other men. In fact, moderate and heavy drinking actually increased the risk of death, with heavy drinking defined as three or more drinks daily. British researchers published those findings in the April 2000 issue of *Heart*.

The most important question, of course, is should *you* drink? Yes, the data supporting the notion of light to moderate alcohol consumption offering protection keeps piling up. One of the most recent reports, in the *British Medical Journal* in 2000, estimated that the average individual can lower the overall risk of CHD by nearly 25 percent by having one drink a day, or perhaps a little more.

Most authorities now agree that those who regularly indulge in a drink or two a day should not be encouraged to stop. Conversely, virtually no one would encourage those who do not currently drink to start doing so in hopes of protecting his or her heart. So unless you have contraindications to alcohol use, the decision is yours. And, as always, if you have any question about that decision, talk to your personal physician about it.

5
Antioxidants, Supplements, and Your Heart

I guess it was a matter of dumb luck when I made my own decision to supplement my heart-healthy diet with antioxidants. Although many advocates had sung the praises of vitamins C and E and beta-carotene for years, back in 1984 there wasn't much in the way of association with heart disease. But since my goal was good health and longevity, I started swallowing a few pills daily though I made no mention of this in *The 8-Week Cholesterol Cure*. That was then, this is now.

Traditionally, purists have chanted the dogma that a balanced diet containing a wide variety of foods provides all the vitamins, minerals, and other nutrients needed for good health. At most, they would grudgingly concede, taking a one-a-day supplement as "insurance" does no harm.

They point as evidence to the recommended dietary allowances (RDAs) for nutrients determined by the National Research Council/ National Academy of Sciences. In truth, those RDAs were amounts needed to prevent deficiency states. Eat too few foods rich in vitamin C, for example, and run the risk of developing scurvy. A niacin deficiency could lead to pellagra.

Now, I ask you: When was the last time you or your doctor encountered such deficiencies? Sure, the average diet can provide minimum levels of nutrients known to prevent disorders not seen since the days English sailors went off to sea with little more to eat than salt pork and crackers. But the better question is not "What is the minimum we need?" but "What is the optimum level for maximal health benefits?"

Even today, however, I can understand how doctors and other health authorities can be easily turned off by wild, unsupported claims made by supplement peddlers. Exaggeration appears to be the norm. "Our supplements are superior because they're made from ingredients grown in Timbuktu!" "Our advanced formulations were developed by an award-winning researcher!" Most such claims are pure bunk. Sadly, they cloud the true picture coming out of major research institutes.

How do we arrive at scientific proof providing certainty to a concept that begins as a theory? Despite the notions of breakthroughs touted in a newspaper today and forgotten tomorrow, the process is neither rapid nor precisely defined. The picture of scientific truth does not suddenly appear. Rather, it emerges in bits and pieces more akin to a mosaic formed out of shards of colored glass.

One research study provides this bit of information. The next project reveals a little more. Sometimes the bits and pieces can, if viewed separately, seem frustratingly contradictory. Yet, over a period of time a clearer picture appears.

Commonly, controversy rages when new ideas are presented. Positions are taken on both sides of a scientific argument. Does washing one's hands before surgery help prevent infection? Are worms created by animal hairs dropping into water? Does the earth revolve around the sun or the sun around the earth? Viewed years later, such disputes seem laughably simple. Yet the scientific process moves forward with excruciatingly slow steps. Sometimes people on the wrong side of the argument give advice that's ultimately proven to be harmful.

So when a decision must be made regarding a course of action that may or may not ultimately be beneficial, one must ask if any harm might be done by making the wrong choice. In the case of dietary supplements, the decision seems to be relatively simple. As we'll see in the coming pages, there seems to be some evidence that supplementation will do our hearts great benefit while virtually everyone agrees that such supplements can do no harm at levels typically recommended. Doctors call this analysis a risk-benefit ratio, and in my mind there have been few instances in which the risk is so small or nonexistent while the benefit potential is so great.

As a person formally trained as a scientist and journalist, I tend to be doubly skeptical about things. And I love to have absolute, unequivocal evidence. Should I take those supplements or not? How many milligrams of this or that?

But what sort of study would it take to deliver that kind of certainty? The perfect study would involve many thousands of men and women of various ages, races, and environmental conditions. Ideally they should all be similar if not identical in lifestyle decisions that could influence outcomes. Participants would be tracked over time and half of them would be given placebos. Those getting the supplements would be further divided into those getting, say, vitamin E, or vitamin C, or selenium, or vitamin A, or combinations and permutations of each. Sounds difficult and expensive? You bet. It will never happen.

So what to do? We take a close look at the emerging picture being formed from hundreds of research investigations that have already been conducted, place most of our trust in studies published in trustworthy medical journals by highly trained scientists with excellent credentials, and disregard claims made by those with vested interests.

A review of the medical literature reveals one undeniable fact. There are vastly more studies showing a positive benefit from antioxidant consumption, from both foods and supplements, than there are negative findings. At the other end of the spectrum, only two studies found a harmful effect. That was a peculiar link between supplementation with beta-carotene and lung cancer incidence; even then, only smokers were affected. No one really understands how beta-carotene might increase a smoker's risk, but that appears to be the statistical fact.

The weird part about the beta-carotene enigma is that most supplements on the market contain an amount of beta-carotene, a precursor to vitamin A, that is relatively small in comparison with that available from foods such as carrots and sweet potatoes. Yet no one cautions against eating too much of these foods. Actually, it's so easy to get plenty of beta-carotene—along with the literally hundreds of chemical cousins collectively called carotenoids—that, for most people, a normal diet will provide enough.

That's not true for other antioxidants, however. Vitamin E comes from just a few foods including vegetable oils and nuts, in relatively small quantities per serving. But the only way to obtain the doses recommended in research studies touting the benefits of vitamin E is through supplements. The same holds true for vitamin C. You can get a lot from orange juice, bell peppers, and other foods, but it would be difficult to achieve potentially valuable dosage levels without consuming excessive calories. And when it comes to selenium, produce from many parts of the country is deficient in this mineral owing to low selenium levels in the soil.

Even with all that in mind, however, you should be aware that many studies have shown the benefits of antioxidants based on blood levels attained just by consuming a heart-healthy diet, which includes plenty of fruits and vegetables. One could argue, therefore, that dietary improvements alone are sufficient. But this assumption would be based on only part of the research published to date. Many other studies employed supplements, at dosage levels virtually impossible to achieve with diet alone.

Some researchers have advocated supplemental antioxidants for decades. That advice was based on the ability of certain nutrients to control levels of free radicals in the blood. Free radicals are chemical entities, principally oxygen, that in a potentially reactive state can be harmful.

In simple terms, free-radical oxidation in the body may be compared to the rusting of an iron pipe in the presence of moisture and oxygen. Some believe that most of the body's degeneration and aging can be attributed to free-radical oxidation. That degeneration may lead to forms of cancer, arthritis, physical deterioration, and of course, heart disease.

About 20 years ago, doctors made the observation that LDL, the bad cholesterol, was formed into arterial plaque only after oxidation. They hypothesized that if oxidation could be prevented by way of antioxidants, LDL and Lp(a) would be less dangerous and less likely to promote clogging of the coronary arteries.

One of the leading research centers for antioxidant investigation is the Texas Southwestern Medical Center in Dallas. There, Dr. Ishwarlal "Kenny" Jialal laid the foundation for vitamin E's ability to prevent LDL oxidation. In a study he presented in the medical literature and at scientific symposia, Dr. Jialal explained that 800 IUs of vitamin E reduced oxidation by 62 percent. He also found that beta-carotene could prevent LDL from being sucked into the gooey muck that forms the atherosclerotic plaque.

Publishing in the American Heart Association's official *Circulation* in 1994, Dr. Jialal wrote of 36 healthy male volunteers who were given a vitamin "cocktail" consisting of 800 IUs of vitamin E, 1000 mg of vitamin C, and 30 mg of beta-carotene. The oxidation of LDL was effectively prevented.

Very importantly, neither Dr. Jialal nor other doctors have ever found any toxicity or adverse reactions to those antioxidant dosages in supplement form. I'll go into more detail on the safety issue shortly.

As any reputable scientist will tell you, one study, or even two, does not necessarily prove a concept to be true. The acid test for truth is termed "reproducibility": Do other researchers get the same results when the concept is tested in their laboratories? The antioxidant theory passed that test with flying colors.

At the University of Minnesota's School of Public Health, laboratory studies of blood samples from ten volunteers who took 800 IUs of vitamin E daily for just two weeks showed up to a threefold increase in their LDL cholesterol's resistance to oxidation. As Dr. John Belcher reported in the journal *Arteriosclerosis and Thrombosis*, elevated levels of vitamin E in the blood appeared to prevent or reduce the toxicity of oxidized LDL, that is, its ability to injure the endothelial cells that line blood vessel walls.

Benefits of antioxidants have been demonstrated for both men and women. The Nurses' Health Study is a long-term project involving more than 87,000 women aged 34 to 59 years of age from across the United States. Over the course of eight years, 17 percent of the nurses took vitamin E supplements at least some of the time. During that time, 552 cases of heart attacks were diagnosed in the test group. But after adjusting for age, smoking, obesity, exercise, and other risk factors, the nurses who took vitamin E had only two-thirds the risk of cardiovascular disease compared with those not taking the supplements. Women who took vitamin E for more than two years had about half the risk.

Meir Stampfer, at Harvard's School of Public Health, was one of the principal investigators in the Nurses' Health Study. The results pleasantly surprised even him. It's worth quoting him from an interview done at the time the study was presented at an AHA meeting:

I'm skeptical by nature but I was even more skeptical going into this study. It just didn't seem plausible that a simple maneuver like taking vitamin E would have such a profound effect. So even though there was a lot of sound scientific basis for the hypothesis that antioxidant vitamins can reduce heart disease, I expected to show that this was not in fact a true association.

A parallel study was performed with participants in the ongoing Health Professionals Follow-Up Study involving nearly 46,000 men aged 40 to 75. Again, after adjusting for major cardiovascular disease risk factors, men who had taken vitamin E for more than two years had a 26 percent lower risk of heart disease than those not taking the vitamin. Those taking the most vitamin E also had a significant reduction in overall mortality. Benefits of taking beta-carotene were also seen.

The following year—1995—researchers at the University of Southern California reported that antioxidant vitamin intake reduced the progression of coronary artery atherosclerosis, as demonstrated by angiograms taken of the actual coronary arteries. Patients received both vitamins E and C.

Scarcely a month goes by in which there isn't more evidence piled onto the heap. Even the normally conservative *Harvard Heart Letter* of August 1997 said that "most research focusing on high dose supplements suggests that this strategy may well provide protection against coronary artery disease. . . . The evidence supporting vitamin E is compelling."

In the fall of 2000, a rather unusual and interesting study published in *Free Radical Biology and Medicine* showed that those having a heart attack whose blood levels of vitamin E were high suffered less heart muscle damage than those with lower levels of the nutrient. Thus, even those for whom vitamin E wasn't sufficient to completely remove MI risk were still somewhat protected.

It appears that vitamin E does even more than prevent the oxidation of harmful LDL molecules. Research presented in April 2000, from Boston University, showed vitamin E's ability to render blood platelets less sticky and likely to form clots. Dr. Jialal from Texas announced that vitamin E also prevents white blood cells from forming plaque by acting as an anti-inflammatory agent. And Tufts University researchers revealed that vitamin E affects the way a variety of cells circulating in our blood interact with artery walls, lessening damage and resultant inflammation.

But it's not just vitamin E alone. Vitamin C has a beneficial effect on the lining of arteries as well, protecting them from damage. The two vitamins also seem to work as a team, each reinforcing the actions of the other, synergizing the beneficial effects. In fact, it's far more than a cumulative effect; the whole is greater than the sum of its parts.

Amid the literally hundreds of published antioxidant studies, it's not surprising that some come up with negative results. The HOPE study found no benefit for individuals previously diagnosed with heart disease. But perhaps the study would have shown protection over a longer period of time, or for those whose hearts were not already badly damaged. At the University of Washington, vitamins C and E were seen to "blunt" the HDL-raising and triglyceride-lowering effects of a combination therapy of statin drugs and niacin. But no other study ever found such an effect. I personally experimented with the concept, removing antioxidants from my own regimen for a while, and found no correlation whatever. Bear in mind that the *vast* majority of published reports have shown cardiovascular protection from antioxidants, both in the diet and from supplements.

As prelude to what I'm about to tell you next, keep in mind that I do not advocate eating heavy, high-fat meals. Such meals reduce the ability of arteries to dilate properly. Yet one study showed that taking vitamins E and C prior to a high-fat meal prevented that arterial impairment, thus offering protection. However, high-fat meals still raise levels of triglycerides and fibrinogen, which make the blood more prone to clotting.

So we have quite a lot of solid, well-documented evidence that vitamins E and C and beta-carotene provide heart-healthy benefits. Studies also show that the mineral selenium acts as a very powerful antioxidant. In addition to eating a heart-smart diet loaded with fruits and vegetables of all sorts, there are plenty of reasons to supplement the diet with vitamin E, vitamin C, some beta-carotene, and selenium.

Personally, I take 600 IUs of vitamin E daily, 300 in the morning and another 300 later in the day. I also supplement my diet with 500 mg of vitamin C in a sustained-release formulation twice daily. My vitamin E supplement contains 6 mg of beta-carotene, and I get a lot more than that from my diet. I happen to love carrot juice, which is loaded with carotenoids in general and beta-carotene in particular. Finally I get 200 µg of selenium daily by way of food and supplements.

No doubt there are a number of companies that manufacture high-quality vitamin and mineral supplements, but sadly many fall short. Laboratory evaluations have revealed that some supplements do not contain the amount of a given nutrient listed on the label. Others have tremendous variation in quality. Some do not dissolve properly in the digestive tract and are not bioavailable.

In virtually all other instances, whether a nutrient comes from a natural source or is manufactured in a factory makes no difference: the body recognizes and uses that nutrient just the same. But that's not the case for vitamin E.

The natural form, listed on labels as d-alpha-tocopherol, is more potent and preferred by the body than the synthetic form, dl-alpha-tocopherol. Watch out for that *l*. Natural E is up to 50 percent more active, so even though it may be more expensive, it's worth it. Most products are synthetic, even those listed as "natural," since companies can get away with that label claim if the product has mixed tocopherols, both natural and synthetic.

The company whose products I use is Endurance Products in Tigard, Oregon, just outside of Portland. I do not own any stock in the company, nor do I receive any benefit for recommending their products. I've been very pleased with all their supplements, find them to be of the highest possible quality and uniformity, like the notion of their sustained-release formulations, and am delighted that the prices are among the lowest you can find anywhere. That's because the company does no advertising; most of its business is done in manufacturing products sold nationally by companies under those companies' own labels. The vitamin E product, called Beta-Cal-E, contains only natural vitamin E. If you'd like to have the same supplements I use daily, which I've been taking successfully since 1988, you can call for an order form at 800-483-2532. Or visit their Web site at www.endur.com. Note that their Endur-VM multivitamin-mineral supplement contains 150 µg of selenium, so there's no need to buy the mineral separately if you choose that particular one.

OTHER REASONS TO SUPPLEMENT WITH ANTIOXIDANTS

All of us want to avoid heart disease and heart attacks. Antioxidants just might give us a bit of an edge against this nasty killer of men and women. But there's evidence that supplements may do our bodies good in a number of other ways.

Take vitamin E. Finnish researchers reported in 1998 that it may prevent prostate cancer. Those taking just 50 IUs daily for five to eight years had a 32 percent lower rate than men who did not take the supplement. Vitamin E may also delay the progression of Alzheimer's disease, as published in the April 1997 issue of the *New England Journal of Medicine*. A study at Tufts University found supplementation improved the immune system in elderly subjects. Moreover, studies by the National Institute of Aging point to slowing of the aging process with vitamin E.

Combining vitamin E with vitamin C paid off big-time for another group studied by the National Institute on Aging. Deaths from all causes in general and from coronary heart disease were reduced in those taking the two supplements. While vitamin E alone cut risk, benefits were improved by adding vitamin C.

In the June 1999 issue of the *American Journal of Nutrition*, a group of researchers advocated that the RDA of vitamin C be doubled to 120 mg. Why? Because greater intake has been associated with reduced risk of chronic diseases, including cancer, heart disease, and cataracts. One of the authors, Dr. Balz Frei, was particularly adamant and effusive, saying, "It's quite amazing how consistent the data on this are."

But how much vitamin C is enough? Beyond 200 mg, the critics like to point out, the body excretes the vitamin in the urine. However, a saturated blood level does not reveal the amount in the tissues where vitamin C confers its health benefits. And such benefits have been shown with up to 1000 mg daily. Moreover, there is absolutely no risk of any side effects from 1000 mg of vitamin C per day.

Next we come to selenium. Researchers at Cornell University were disappointed at first that the trace mineral had no effect on the incidence of skin cancer as they had hoped. But total cancer incidence and mortality owing to cancer of the lung, prostate, and colon were all decreased by about half. Participants in the study were given 200 micrograms (μg) of selenium daily for several years.

Can selenium supplementation achieve such spectacular results for everyone? It all depends on the amount of the trace element already in the diet. And the problem is that most of us have no idea as to the amount of our intake. As stated earlier, some areas of the country have particularly selenium-poor soil, and crops grown in that soil won't provide the nutrient. It seems wise to get that little extra insurance through selenium supplementation. But don't go over the 200 μg dosage. First of all, more than that doesn't really do any good, and second, doses of 1000 μg or more lead to side effects, including hair and fingernail loss. If one persists in taking such high doses, the results can be lethal. But that said, 200 μg is completely safe.

I believe that as the years go by, scientists will discover more and more benefits to dietary supplementation. Eventually supplements will be recommended by doctors for virtually everyone.

IS ONE ANTIOXIDANT BEST?

All the antioxidants discussed in this chapter have been found to protect against heart disease in one way or another. Certainly vitamin E has gotten the lion's share of research attention. If one had to choose only one antioxidant to include in a heart-healthy regimen, I'd have to give the nod to vitamin E, especially in its natural form. The dosage range for optimum heart-related benefits appears to be 400 to 800 IUs.

But why stop there? Vitamin E does its best work when accompanied by vitamin C, which also prevents breakdown of vitamin E. And vitamin C definitely has a positive effect on the arteries' ability to dilate for greater blood flow by maintaining elasticity of the endothelial lining.

Selenium, too, cooperates with vitamin E in protecting against LDL oxidation. But the role of this trace element is a bit different from that of the other antioxidants. It defends the endothelial cell lining of arteries against the assault of oxidized LDL and also increases production of prostacyclin, a hormone-like substance that protects the heart while inhibiting production of thromboxane, which has been strongly implicated in the development of atherosclerotic plaque. Niacin also offers this particular benefit.

Finally we come to beta-carotene. Once the darling of supplementation advocates, this antioxidant's glow has dimmed. That's because of the unexplained association between beta-carotene supplementation and incidence of lung cancer in smokers. It would seem more logical to me, however, to strongly counsel smokers to quit their habit rather than point the finger at beta-carotene.

Fortunately, it's pretty easy to get lots of beta-carotene in a balanced diet. But bear in mind that there are dozens of research articles underscoring beta-carotene's heart-protective qualities.

I wouldn't go out of my way to take a single-nutrient beta-carotene supplement tablet. That's especially because beta-carotene is just one of several hundred carotenoids in foods. I'd rather eat a few carrots or drink a glass of carrot juice. On the other hand, a bit of beta-carotene supplementation can certainly do no harm and just might do some good.

CONVERTING MEASUREMENTS OF VITAMIN E AND BETA-CAROTENE

Vitamin C, also known as ascorbic acid, is always listed in milligrams (mg) on foods and supplements. But beta-carotene can be measured either in milligrams or international units (IUs). One mg of beta-carotene equals 1667 IUs. Thus 25,000 IU contains 15 mg.

Vitamin E is most often measured in IUs, but now and then you will see it in milligrams. Conversion depends on the form of vitamin E involved. Natural d-alpha-tocopherol converts as 1.49 IUs per mg when it is in the succinate form. Natural vitamin E in its acetate form converts as 1.36 IUs per mg. For synthetic acetate— dl-alpha-tocopherol—the equation is 1.0 IU to 1.0 mg. You might also see "mixed tocopherols" on a label, in which case figure 1.25 IUs per mg.

THE DECISION IS YOURS

I've been taking antioxidant supplements since 1984. The intervening years have yielded volumes of validation for that decision. How much of my own heart health can I attribute to those tablets? I really don't know. But I do know this: I feel the research data that antioxidants help protect the heart are so compelling that there's no way anyone could convince me to stop taking them. Should you also take them?

Don't for a minute think that antioxidant tablets are a replacement for fruits, vegetables, and whole grains in your diet. They are supplements and not replacements. I cannot emphasize that too much.

Don't rely on antioxidants to ease your conscience if you refuse to maintain regular, fairly strenuous physical activity or fight the ill effects of smoking.

The decision to supplement with antioxidants should be one of completing a full program of heart-healthy lifestyle. And, as in everything, the ultimate decision is yours.

6
Yup, Oat Bran Really Works

The journey of a thousand miles, they say, begins with a single step. For me, the first step toward my own cholesterol control was the finding that the soluble fiber in oat bran could bring cholesterol levels down.

I knew that simply avoiding high-fat foods didn't do the trick. Perhaps there were foods that could actually be good for the heart.

Coincidentally, I had met Dr. David Kritchevsky of the Wistar Institute at the University of Pennsylvania in Philadelphia while doing an interview in the mid-1970s. He found that feeding rabbits lots of alfalfa brought their cholesterol counts down, even when they were fed a high-fat diet. But people aren't rabbits and most of us wouldn't want much alfalfa in our diets.

Doing a literature review, using the keywords "fiber" and "cholesterol," I stumbled on the work of Dr. James Anderson at the University of Kentucky. Dr. Anderson was doing a systematic study to determine if one cereal was better than another in controlling blood sugar. Lo and behold, oats were the winner. He also noted, rather coincidentally, that cholesterol levels came down as well.

But what was it about oats that got the job done? Anyone who has ever cooked up a pot of oatmeal knows about the gel that forms on the sides of the pot. The best way to clean up that pot is to soak it in cold water. The gel, you'll remember, swells and can then be easily removed. It turns out that the gel, which contains a type of soluble fiber called beta-glucan, is the magic ingredient.

While oats are an excellent source of soluble fiber, that fiber is particularly concentrated in the bran fraction of the whole-oat grain. In fact, it takes 1½ cups of oatmeal to provide the same amount of beta-glucan in 1 cup of oat bran.

Since I prefer oat bran muffins to hot cereal, I made three muffins a day a part of my cholesterol-lowering experimental regimen, which also included a low-fat diet and the vitamin niacin. Eight weeks later, bingo! My total cholesterol fell from 284 to 169. The rest, as they say, is history.

But the resulting book stirred up quite a bit of controversy here in the United States and around the world. Some questioned the true effectiveness of a mere cereal in cholesterol control. Others complained that people wouldn't be able to eat enough to have any significant effect. In Australia, scientists wondered if oat bran Down Under would have the same benefits as the American version.

One by one, those concerns were put to rest. Numerous studies documented oat bran's cholesterol-lowering properties. It didn't take enough oats to, as one newsletter punned, "choke a horse" to see benefits. And indeed, Australian oat bran was just as good as the American grain.

More to the point, readers learned that oat bran really worked. They wrote letters telling me of their success and they told their friends and neighbors. The resulting word of mouth made the book the biggest-selling health book of the 1980s. In fact, because of that book, the world faced an oat bran shortage!

Fads come and go. But this was more than just a dietary fad. As a result, the U.S. Food and Drug Administration allowed manufacturers to make the first health claim ever for oats.

Sadly, there was one badly flawed study that got lots of media attention in the late 1980s. Basing their conclusions on an extremely small group of female health professionals whose cholesterol levels were normal to begin with, the researchers said oat bran worked no better than the fiber-free Cream of Wheat.

The story of the cereal killers has become a classic. As recently as late 1994 students at the Wistar Institute studied the episode in a seminar dealing with science, politics, and public policy. Even undergraduate students were able to poke holes in the flawed study and wondered how it all could have happened.

A more careful analysis of the research authors' own data demonstrate oat bran's effectiveness, rather than denying it. They claimed that everything was equal in both the oat bran (OB) and Cream of Wheat (CW) groups, but a closer look shows that is not true. The OB group consumed a diet in which 35 percent of calories came from fat while the CW group's diet contained only 30 percent fat. In truth, it was remarkable that oat bran consumption would allow all those extra grams of fat to be enjoyed while keeping cholesterol levels low.

The authors also claimed that there were no differences in

cholesterol levels between the two groups. But that was true only for total cholesterol. Eating the low-fat, high-carbohydrate diet, the CW group experienced a decline in HDL from an average of 54 down to 50.9. Conversely, the OB group had a slight increase from the initial average of 54 to 54.2 for HDL readings.

That difference in HDL translates to a distinct improvement in the risk ratio of TC to HDL for the OB group. The CW group's risk worsened.

But because the researchers were from Harvard University and were backed by the massive public relations brawn of the Center for Science in the Public Interest, which had a vendetta against the Quaker Oats Company, the publicity surge was huge. Comedians made jokes on late-night TV about the fall of oat bran. Sales fell. Like Humpty Dumpty, no one could put confidence in oat bran back together again.

PROOF KEEPS PILING UP

Literally dozens of papers were published demonstrating the cholesterol-lowering might of oats and oat bran in general, and the beta-glucan soluble fiber in particular. Here's a sampling.

In 1991, Dr. Anderson saw a 12.8 percent drop in TC and a 12.1 percent drop in LDL after 21 days of consuming 110 grams of oat bran daily. That's about 4 ounces. That same year New Zealand workers found an 11.6 percent TC decline with a rise of 10.3 percent in HDL in those eating almost 2 ounces of oat bran cooked into muffins daily for four weeks. In Chicago, noted nutrition researcher Dr. Linda Van Horn demonstrated a 6.25 percent drop in TC and a 9.2 percent drop in LDL after eight weeks of consuming 2 ounces of instant oats.

German researchers in 1992 found that about 2 ounces of oat bran daily brought TC down by 9.7 percent in just three weeks. Australians that same year reported a 5.7 percent decline in LDL and a 7.5 percent improvement in the LDL-HDL ratio in subjects consuming about 2 ounces of oat bran as muffins.

The findings continued to come in. In 1993, a Louisiana State University study showed a 10 percent reduction in TC with a 13.5 percent fall in LDL in three weeks of eating 4 ounces of oat bran. That same amount achieved an 8.2 percent decline in TC and a 9.9 percent drop in LDL, as reported in the *Journal of the American Dietetic Association* in 1994.

BUT HOW DOES IT WORK?

I was first impressed by the potential of oat bran back in the mid-1980s when I realized that its mode of action was similar, if not identical, to prescription drugs called resins, used to lower cholesterol. Both act as "bile-sequestering agents."

The liver uses cholesterol to make bile acids, which are necessary in the digestive process. Unused bile gets recycled, but when you eat oats, the soluble fiber forms a gel in the digestive tract that binds onto bile, eliminating it with the bowel movement. Picture this as a glacier moving through your gut, removing cholesterol as it passes through. Since bile contains cholesterol, and the bile is removed, the body must make more. To do so, it takes cholesterol out of the bloodstream. We know that oat bran actually gets rid of that bile, and hence the cholesterol, because researchers have literally measured the amounts in the feces—not a pleasant job but someone had to do it.

Soluble fiber may also have a second mechanism of action. It is fermented in the colon to form certain kinds of fatty acids, which are absorbed by a vein in the abdomen and then transported directly to the liver, where they inhibit cholesterol manufacture.

Soluble fiber also helps us control weight in two ways. First, it stabilizes the level of sugars in the bloodstream. As a result, blood sugar doesn't drop as quickly and one doesn't get hungry for quite a while after a soluble fiber–rich meal. Second, it promotes a feeling of satisfaction, termed satiety, owing to the slow movement of the gel formed by the soluble fiber with water as it passes through the digestive system.

So soluble fiber works. We can realistically expect results from this single element in a heart-smarter lifestyle because studies from all over the world, working with a wide variety of foods and supplements, have shown cholesterol reductions from as low as 3 percent to as much as 25 percent. More typically, drops are in the 9 to 11 percent range.

Both total cholesterol and LDL cholesterol come down when soluble fibers are added into the diet. But it's critical to note that the levels of protective HDL cholesterol do not drop. Now that is quite different from the effects of a commonly advocated low-fat, high-carbohydrate diet, which inevitably results in a significant HDL decline along with a rise in triglycerides. By keeping the HDL up and getting total and LDL cholesterols down, a low-fat diet with added soluble fibers is much more effective in improving the vital risk ratio of TC to HDL and LDL to HDL than a standard low-fat diet.

Moreover, you will find it a whole lot easier to add something to the diet than to subtract it.

I noted that cholesterol improvements vary considerably from study to study. Those with high numbers to begin with will do best. But as a rule of thumb you can figure on about a 5 percent cholesterol reduction by consuming 3 grams daily of soluble fiber. To get that amount, you would need $^1/_2$ cup of uncooked oat bran (1 cup cooked) or $^3/_4$ cup of uncooked oatmeal. But oats are just one of the many sources of soluble fiber; other sources include barley, beans, psyllium, figs, and various supplements. The trick is to include all those foods in your diet so you never get tired of eating just one thing day after day.

BEANS, BEANS, GOOD FOR YOUR HEART

One easy way to get lots of soluble fiber into the diet is by eating a variety of dried beans and peas. Research has shown that 1 cup of beans provides the cholesterol-lowering effect of $^1/_2$ cup of oat bran. And as with oat bran, studies have indicated cholesterol reductions of anywhere from 3 to 10 percent or more. Importantly, only the bad LDL goes down, leaving the protective HDL levels intact. Of all the dried beans and peas, one of the richest sources of soluble fiber is black-eyed peas. Try them out of a can, drained and rinsed, or prepare them from scratch. For a real treat, look for fresh black-eyed peas in your supermarket's produce section. Simmer the peas in water for about 15 minutes and serve with a drizzle of extra-virgin olive oil—you'll experience one more example of the ultrahealthy Mediterranean diet.

Think about the variety of beans: pinto beans in chili, white beans in soup, refried beans in Mexican meals, Cuban-style black beans with roasted chicken and rice. And then there are red beans in Cajun cooking, kidney beans in minestrone, three-bean salads, hummus, that staple of Middle Eastern cuisine made out of chickpeas (garbanzo beans). The list goes on and on.

Concerned about gas? Don't cook the beans in the same water used for soaking, and consider trying Beano when you eat beans. The product is very effective in preventing the formation of gas from undigested beans fermenting in the digestive tract.

Like oat bran, beans really work. In one study Dr. Anderson, who has studied beans extensively, found that a daily cup of vegetarian pork and beans cut cholesterol levels by 13 percent. The men in his study made no other dietary changes, continuing to eat a standard diet that was 38 percent fat. He believes that while canned beans are good, dried beans appear to be better. His study produced a whopping 19 percent reduction in cholesterol counts with dried beans.

A BOWL OF BARLEY

Barley was once a staple in American cooking. Today consumption has declined, but you should consider adding it back to your shopping list as an excellent source of fiber and nutrition. Researchers in Minnesota and North Dakota learned that barley is an excellent alternative to oat bran in the fight against cholesterol and heart disease.

At the University of Minnesota, Dr. Joseph Keenan found that barley had a significant positive effect on satiety in 60 overweight men and women, helping them in their efforts to lose those extra pounds. At the same time, total cholesterol fell by 11 percent and LDL by 12 percent. Dr. Keenan provided 7 grams of beta-glucan to subjects daily by way of barley muffins. Those getting ordinary wheat muffins did not derive the same benefits. He reported his findings at the Experimental Biology 2000 meeting.

While ordinary barley does offer a cholesterol-lowering effect, a newly developed strain of the grain does far more. The so-called waxy, hull-less barley developed at North Dakota State University contains two to three times as much beta-glucan as normal barley. The new barley is also rich in a chemical cousin of vitamin E— d-alpha-tocotrienol—which works in the liver to actually inhibit cholesterol manufacture. Barley gives you a healthy double whammy!

NuWorld Nutrition in Fargo, North Dakota, produces the new barley in a form that can be made into a very satisfying hot cereal. The company also provides recipes for cookies, muffins, and pancakes. Currently this special barley is available only through mail order, but unlike most other mail-order products, this one is quite inexpensive. You can call NuWorld at 800-950-3188 to place an order.

BRAN, SEEDS, AND PECTIN

Other types of bran have similar cholesterol-lowering capabilities. Both corn bran and rice bran have racked up data demonstrating their effectiveness. In 1993, for example, researchers from Louisiana State University published findings that rice bran was as effective as oat bran in cholesterol control.

Neither type of bran, however, attained the popularity of oat bran, and you might have trouble finding either one. Look for them in stores and supermarkets specializing in health foods. You'll probably have an easier time finding flaxseed, which also has a cholesterol-lowering characteristic. Research published in the *Journal of the American College of Nutrition* showed a 10 percent cholesterol reduction after eating flaxseed-enriched bread for two months. Flaxseed is also a good source of omega-3 fatty acids, the kind found in fish, which protect against excessive formation of blood clots.

Next we come to pectin, another type of soluble fiber found in apples. While an apple contains only a small amount of pectin, you can find a concentrated form that can be deliciously incorporated into a variety of baked goods such as cookies, muffins, and cakes. Use it to replace an equal amount of flour in your recipes. You can order pectin from Tastee Apple Fiber at 800-262-7753.

While you're on the phone with your credit card out, you may wish to place an order for a concentrated form of oat bran fiber. Developed originally by a division of the U.S. Department of Agriculture, oatrim, sold under the brand name Beta-Trim by Bob's Red Mill Natural Foods, is a wonderful product with many uses.

Since soluble fiber absorbs and holds fluids, it acts as a natural fat replacer in baked goods. You can cut fat in recipes by half. And here's a way to make your hamburgers juicier. Start with ultra-low-fat ground beef, mix in some oatrim as you might use breadcrumbs, along with beef broth. The oatrim will absorb and hold the broth, adding flavor and juiciness to the burgers. Try this also with your meatloaf and meatball recipes. Bob's Red Mill sells oatrim in 16- and 32-ounce packages. Call 503-654-3215 in Milwaukee.

PSYLLIUM: A SERIOUS CHOLESTEROL FIGHTER

Psyllium is a particularly concentrated form of soluble fiber derived from the seed husks of a plant grown in arid regions. The most common source is Metamucil and similar products, sold mainly as laxatives. For those already regular, additions of psyllium to the daily diet will not act as a purgative. In fact, psyllium is often prescribed by physicians for those battling chronic diarrhea, acting by absorbing excess fluid in the colon. Bran Buds, Kellogg's all-bran cereal, contains a good amount of psyllium. The good news is that psyllium provides a very efficient, effective method of cholesterol control.

In one of the early studies with this fiber, Dr. James Anderson gave participants 3.4 grams of psyllium three times daily with meals. That's the amount found in one rounded teaspoon of Metamucil, which is mixed into water or juice. Twenty-six men followed the program, which had no other change in diet, for eight weeks. Total cholesterol fell by nearly 15 percent, and LDL counts came down by about 20 percent. A study using just over 5 grams of psyllium yielded about a 6 percent reduction. Research published in 1998 and in 2000 replicated those positive findings.

To maximize the effects of psyllium on cholesterol reduction, it's best to have it close to meal times. Always mix it in a large glass of water or juice; ironically, soluble fiber of any kind can have a consti-pating effect if fluid intake is insufficient. And it would be far better to have the total dosage divided throughout the day; three 1-teaspoon doses would be more effective than one 1-tablespoon dose.

Caution! Don't be fooled by advertisements for non-psyllium look-alike products. Citrucel, for example, compares itself directly with Metamucil, citing its superior solubility, taste, and texture. Although both are high-fiber supplements that promote regularity, Citrucel contains methylcellulose, not psyllium, and has *no effect* on cholesterol reduction. Although it dissolves in water, Citrucel is not a soluble fiber. Soluble fibers, by their nature and definition, form a gel when mixed with water.

When buying the Kellogg's cereal, be sure the label has the desig-nation "Bran Buds" since there are other varieties of all-bran cereals on the market. Always check the ingredients list for psyllium.

FRUITS AND VEGGIES FOR FIBER

I don't think vegetarians are healthier because they don't eat meat, but rather, because they eat a lot of fruits and vegetables. Lacto-ovo vegetarians, for example consume dairy foods and eggs, yet they share the same benefits as those who avoid animal products entirely.

Throughout this book you will read about the advantages of fruits and vegetables. They're a great source of antioxidants—the best, in fact. They contain flavonoids. In addition, they probably have beneficial chemical substances scientists have yet to identify. They deserve a mention in this chapter because they are an excellent source of soluble—as well as insoluble—fiber. For amounts of fiber, see Table 6.

Make a conscious decision to increase your daily intake. Figs and prunes are the real winners in the soluble fiber showdown, so why not have them readily available for munching when watching TV? Or keep some single-serving packets in the glove compartment of your car, in your office drawer, or even in your attaché case, golf bag, and wherever else is convenient.

The Nurses' Health Study has given us a lot of insight into the role of diet in maintaining good health. Some of the latest data show tremendous protection against heart disease for those women who consume the most fiber from fruits, vegetables, and whole-grain cereals.

Table 6. **Finding the Fiber in Foods**

	Total Fiber: g/3.5 oz	Soluble Fiber: g/3.5 oz
Cereals		
All-Bran	30.8	5.1
Barley (regular, pearled)	14.0	3.5
Barley (waxy, hull-less)	18.0	6.5
Bran Buds	36.0	10.0
Cheerios	9.1	4.2
Cream of Wheat (uncooked)	3.8	1.6
Fiber One	42.4	3.0
Oat bran (uncooked)	14.4	7.2
Oat bran (cold cereal)	10.3	5.2
Oat Bran Crunch (Kolln)	16.4	9.3
Oatmeal (uncooked)	9.5	4.9
Raisin Bran	13.5	2.4
Rice Krispies	1.2	0.3
Shredded wheat	12.5	1.6
Wheaties	8.3	2.4
Fruit		
Apple	2.0	0.6
Apricots (dried)	7.9	4.4
Banana	1.9	0.6
Dates (dried)	4.4	1.2
Figs (dried)	8.2	4.0
Orange	2.0	1.0
Pear	3.5	1.3
Prunes (dried)	6.6	3.8
Raisins (dried)	2.3	1.1
Vegetables		
Asparagus	2.0	0.8
Beets	2.6	1.2
Broccoli	3.1	1.5
Brussels sprouts	5.7	3.0
Carrots	3.2	1.5
Cauliflower	1.8	0.9
Corn	2.9	0.5
Potato (sweet)	2.5	1.1

	Total Fiber: g/3.5 oz	Soluble Fiber: g/3.5 oz
Potato (white w/skin)	2.0	1.0
Spinach (cooked)	1.8	0.6
Dried Beans and Peas		
Black beans (cooked)	7.1	2.8
Black-eyed peas (canned)	3.9	0.4
Butter beans (cooked)	7.3	2.9
Chick peas (cooked)	5.3	1.6
Kidney beans (canned)	6.2	1.6
Pinto beans (cooked)	6.9	2.2
Pork and beans (canned)	4.2	2.0
Split peas (cooked)	3.2	1.1
Nuts		
Almonds	8.8	1.1
Peanut butter	6.1	1.6
Sesame seeds	9.1	1.9
Sunflower seeds	6.1	2.1
Walnuts	4.2	1.5
Supplements		
Citrucel (1 tbsp)	2.0	2.0
Citrus pectin (1 tbsp)	5.5	5.5
Flax fiber (2 tbsp)	5.7	2.2
Metamucil (1 tsp)	2.7	2.1
Metamucil, sugar-free (1 tsp)	3.0	2.6
ProFibe (1 scoop)	5.0	5.0

Source: Excerpted by permission from James W. Anderson, *Plant Fiber in Foods,* HCF Nutrition Research Foundation, Lexington, Ky., 1990. Data for some items was drawn from other sources.

Blocking Cholesterol
in the Foods You Love

Do I ever have a wonderful story to tell you! The bottom line, after all the twists and turns, is that there is a completely safe, natural plant substance that can block the absorption of cholesterol from the foods you love to eat but which have been previously forbidden on heart-healthy diets. Today we can enjoy eggs, shrimp, and other cholesterol-rich foods without guilt and without any of the cholesterol getting into our bloodstreams.

Now bear with me as I give you some preliminary information. As you know, saturated fats and trans fats are the real villains in the diet. Those are the components of foods that raise cholesterol levels in the blood the most. Other kinds of fats, we've now learned, don't have a negative effect.

But the other dietary component that can raise cholesterol in the blood is the cholesterol found in animal foods. There's no doubt that dietary cholesterol raises cholesterol in the blood, and thus the risk of heart disease. That's why the AHA and others continue to recommend limits on amounts consumed daily. (See Table 7.)

The link between cholesterol in the diet and in our blood has been reestablished by very recent research. One study looked at the effects of shrimp and eggs. Subjects were asked to eat either 300 grams (10 ounces) of steamed shrimp or two large eggs daily as part of a low-fat diet for a few weeks. The shrimp added 590 mg of cholesterol, and the eggs provided 581 mg.

Shrimp raised LDL cholesterol levels by more than 7 percent; eggs boosted LDL counts by 13 percent. That's a lot, and it really justifies concerns about cholesterol in the diet. And while shrimp and eggs are particularly high in cholesterol, remember that it is present in *all* animal foods, even the leanest cuts of beef and chicken breast.

But here's the interesting thing about those shrimp and eggs. Although LDL levels increased, so did HDL counts. While eating shrimp daily, HDLs went up by more than 12 percent. Daily eggs brought HDLs up by 7.6 percent. That happens to be true for all animal foods.

Now wouldn't it be nice to be able to get the HDL-boosting effects without the LDL increases? That's what happens when the dietary cholesterol is blocked from the bloodstream. And it can be done with a simple plant extract that researchers have been quietly working with for decades.

In my own case, in the ten years following that second bypass operation I did not eat a single egg yolk. I even bought noodles made without yolks, and avoided fresh pasta because of the added eggs. It seemed a small price to pay to keep my blood vessels from clogging, and the egg yolk substitutes were a lot better than when they first came out. But I have to admit that I missed those poached, sunny-side-up, over-easy, boiled, baked, and deviled eggs. There's just no substitute for those yolks!

I had not been alone in my avoidance of eggs and their cholesterol. Egg sales and consumption have plummeted to half their 1960s level. Even the egg industry has tossed in the towel and now recommends the AHA's limit of four eggs a week. Sensitive persons should eat none at all.

While other foods are rich sources of cholesterol, the egg has come to symbolize the deadly dietary component. A very nutritious, inexpensive food that nutritionists use as the gold standard of protein quality has come to be politically incorrect for those wishing to avoid heart disease.

That hits particularly hard in the elderly population. Many older individuals live alone, and meal production becomes a tedious chore. Eggs are the perfect protein source for such men and women. They are inexpensive, easily stored in their own single "packaging," and can be prepared in a wide variety of ways to prevent boredom. Ironically, surveys have shown elderly persons to be undernourished. Yet they avoid eggs because of the cholesterol and their fear of CHD.

But enough of such negatives! Let me start at the beginning.

Cholesterol, of course, is a member of the chemical family called sterols (not steroids), which are present in every animal tissue. Cholesterol is an animal sterol. Plants also contain sterols, which are termed phytosterols. Sort of the yin and yang of nature.

You'll remember that years ago dieticians condemned shellfish for having very high levels of cholesterol. Those early measurements were totally inaccurate because they were counting not only cholesterol but also the phytosterols from the plants those animals ate. Shellfish are the vegetarians of the sea. In truth, certain shellfish have the lowest cholesterol content of any animal food; scallops contain about a third of that found in chicken breast, for example. So do oysters, which my father loved but scrupulously avoided when told they were high in cholesterol. But those early measurement devices just couldn't tell the difference between cholesterol and phytosterol.

Can you tell the difference? Look at the molecular structure shown in Figure 1. *Hint:* look at the little additional "squiggle" at the end of the chain on the phytosterol molecule. The two structures are nearly identical. Didn't see that difference at first?

Well, neither can your body! Cholesterol is absorbed in the first one-third of your intestine by cell receptors called micelles, which then transport it into the bloodstream. Those receptors can't discern between cholesterol and phytosterols, and they'll fill up on whichever happens to be available.

Very early research showed us that the body can absorb only so much cholesterol at a time. Eat three eggs, you might as well eat a dozen. Some gets into a limited number of those specialized cells called micelles, and the rest simply passes through the digestive tract unabsorbed.

So if micelles are filled with phytosterols, they cannot accept cholesterol. Block the cholesterol by filling up the micelles, and that cholesterol passes on through. As we'll see, there's a world of proof for that.

Phytosterols, unlike cholesterol, are not absorbed into the bloodstream. Apparently, that little squiggle of a difference is enough to keep the phytosterols in the micelles for a while—some estimates say an hour or so—and then the micelles, in effect, "spit" the phytosterols out, and they too pass on through the GI tract and out of the body.

Phytosterols are found in all plants, from fruits to vegetables to nuts and seeds. They are particularly concentrated in the plant's oils. You would expect, then, that vegetable oils would be rich sources. But plant sterols cause these oils to be cloudy, and food manufacturers remove them to provide the clear product that consumers prefer. So there is no readily available source of concentrated phytosterols in our diet to balance out the cholesterol.

Interestingly, the Japanese make oil from rice bran, which they remove to produce the white rice they, too, prefer. But they leave the clouding phytosterols in that rice oil. In fact, rice bran oil has been shown to lower cholesterol levels. Maybe that's one reason the Japanese have a low rate of heart disease.

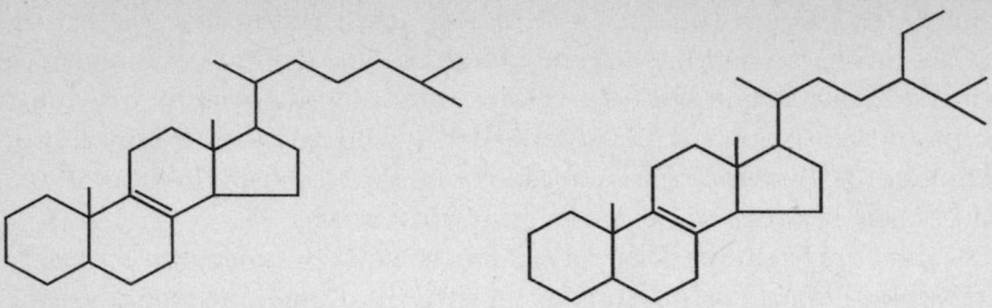

CHOLESTEROL   PHYTOSTEROL

Figure 1
Cholesterol and phytosterol molecules.

The term "phytosterol" is generic; it includes all plant sterols. The principal phytosterols in nature are beta-sitosterol, campesterol, and stigmasterol. Sitosterol is the most potent phytosterol for blocking the absorption of cholesterol. That discovery was first made in the late 1940s at the laboratories of the Upjohn pharmaceutical company in Kalamazoo, Michigan.

During that time, steroid hormones were coming into vogue in the medical community. Cortisone was the miracle drug of its day. Upjohn discovered that those steroid hormones could be made from the soybean sterol stigmasterol. As part of his laboratory investigations at the time, Dr. Drury Petersen fed the soybean sterols to chickens. To his surprise, he found that the chicken's cholesterol levels did not rise, even when fed a cholesterol-rich diet. But Upjohn was not particularly interested in that discovery—they wanted to sell cortisone.

So Upjohn bought crude soybean sterols from food companies such as General Mills, extracted the stigmasterol, and sold the rest, consisting of campesterol and sitosterol, to the Eli Lilly Company in Indiana. Lilly then concocted a cholesterol-lowering drug called Cytellin.

But Cytellin was ahead of its time. Though it did lower cholesterol levels, most people and their doctors were not particularly aware of cholesterol as a risk factor in heart disease. Cytellin had no influence on the effect of fat on blood cholesterol levels; it only blocked the absorption of cholesterol. Moreover, I've heard that it tasted horrible.

Research with phytosterols continued through the 1970s and into the 1980s. Probably the most definitive study came from the laboratories of Drs. Fred Mattson and Scott Grundy, then at the University of California at San Diego. They fed hospitalized patients scrambled eggs and sitosterol and found that the phytosterol blocked absorption of cholesterol, resulting in reduced cholesterol levels in the blood.

Often researchers used phytosterols as a general cholesterol-lowering agent rather than to specifically block the absorption of cholesterol in a particular meal. This meant that sometimes there would be more phytosterol than was needed because there was not much cholesterol in the foods, while at other times there wouldn't be enough to block the absorption of all the cholesterol available. Even so, studies showed total cholesterol reductions of 12 percent on average.

What is exciting about phytosterols is that potentially we can have our cake and eat it too. Using the phytosterols, we can enjoy cholesterol-rich foods while still getting an additional LDL reduction. And by eating those foods, as we've seen earlier, HDL and triglyceride levels go up as well.

In a landmark paper, Drs. Grundy and Mattson concluded that "rather than remove these foods [eggs, etc.] from the diet, the same end could be accomplished by preventing the absorption of cholesterol. Phytosterols have long been known to have this function" (*American Journal of Clinical Nutrition,* April 1982, 697–700).

For quite a while, research interest in the phytosterols died down, though a few papers continued to trickle in. Then researchers in Finland began to study the effects of a slightly modified sterol termed "stanol," from pine tree pulp. The oil from that source is termed "tall oil." And the sterol extracted from the tall oil was chemically altered to make it more easily blended into margarine.

The first Finnish research was published in 1995 in the *New England Journal of Medicine.* For a one-year period, 153 subjects continued with their usual diet and lifestyle and used either regular margarine or a specially prepared margarine laced with the sterols/stanols. Those who ate the stanols lowered their total and LDL cholesterol levels by 11 and 15 percent, respectively, as compared to those consuming the regular margarine.

Quite coincidentally, about two years prior to that, I had been reading all I could find about the phytosterols, and I decided to experiment on myself. That meant eating eggs for the first time in a decade.

Prior to each egg meal—which I relished more than I can express—I swallowed a couple of capsules I'd filled with phytosterol powder I had shipped in from Japan. At the time, there were no phytosterol tablets or capsules on the market. Each of the capsules I'd prepared (thanks to time spent in my dad's pharmacy when I was in high school) contained 400 mg of phytosterols.

To be effective, one has to counteract cholesterol with phytosterols on at least a one-to-one basis. And that's assuming a really high-quality phytosterol preparation. Since one egg contains about 220 mg of cholesterol (extra-large eggs have more), it takes at least that much phytosterol to block its absorption. I took 400 mg for each egg yolk.

Phytosterols in the pure state are a white, slightly waxy substance. They are not soluble in water, so they can't be mixed with orange juice or other beverages. In addition, they must be carefully prepared, since if phytosterols are too tightly packed into capsules or tablets, they may not break up in the digestive tract, where they're supposed to do their job.

For over a month, I ate eggs, shrimp, even low-fat liver sausage, preceding each meal with my phytosterol capsule. Then came the good news. Not only did my LDL level not rise a bit, but my HDLs were up and my triglycerides were down. I knew I was onto something.

Next I convinced some friends to join my experiment, and we all had our cholesterol levels monitored at the office of my close friend and personal physician Dr. Charles Keenan in Santa Monica. Everyone experienced the same results.

But there were no phytosterol products on the market that I could recommend to my readers. So I turned to the company that produces the niacin formulation Endur-acin, which I'd been using and suggesting for years. Terry Hammerschmidt at Endurance Products in Tigard, Oregon, came up with a 400-mg tablet that dissolved in 30 minutes. That meant the tablets had to be taken 30 minutes prior to meals. A bit inconvenient but, considering the benefits, well worth the effort. I told the readers of my *Diet-Heart Newsletter,* and they started into the phytosterols as well. Results were terrific and I received many letters of thanks.

In 1995, I was invited to present a paper on novel approaches to cholesterol control at the International Congress on Heart Health in Barcelona, Spain. There I met the Finnish researchers, before their paper was published in the United States some months later.

The Finnish diet relies heavily on butter or margarine. Practically every meal includes bread with either spread. The Finns eagerly accepted the stanol-laced margarine, marketed to the public under the name Benecol. But I wondered whether Americans would do as well with margarine, since not every meal here calls for it. Moreover, it would be inconvenient to carry one's own margarine to restaurants or on vacation.

The tablets seemed a better bet. But many of the letters I got from readers complained that the timing problem was difficult, and that they forgot to take the tablets prior to meals. There had to be a better way.

Meanwhile, the sterols and stanols got more and more attention in both the scientific literature and the mass media. In a scientific advisory aimed at cardiologists and other physicians and health professionals, the American Heart Association summarized the research documenting the safety and effectiveness of phytosterols in blocking the absorption of dietary cholesterol and in lowering cholesterol levels in the blood. The research was published in the June 1997 issue of *Circulation*.

A year later, Benecol margarine laced with stanols and Take Control margarine with soybean-derived sterols hit the U.S. market.

How much of the spreads would one have to consume to get a cholesterol-lowering effect? In a study of 224 people, those consuming 1 gram (1000 mg) of soy sterols in Take Control margarine daily saw an LDL reduction of 7.6 percent. Increasing the dosage to 2 grams (2000 mg) boosted the effect only to 8.1 percent. The results of that study were presented at the 1999 AHA meeting.

So a dosage of at least 1 gram of sterols daily provides a nice extra cholesterol reduction. But how do the sterols compare with the stanols? For a while, the makers of Benecol margarine claimed that stanols were superior. But a paper published in the December 2000 issue of *American Journal of Clinical Nutrition* found that both sterols and stanols inhibited cholesterol reduction equally, despite their slight chemical differences.

SAFETY OF PHYTOSTEROLS

By this time you have to be wondering about safety and potential side effects. Remarkably, there are no problems, no adverse effects at all. Remember that the phytosterols do not pass into the bloodstream; rather, they are passed with the bowel movement. There is no digestive upset or disturbance of any kind. There are no interactions between phytosterols and either prescribed or over-the-counter drugs or supplements. No other nutrients are blocked or lost. This is an exceptional safety record, documented again and again in the medical literature.

The plant sterols are so safe, in fact, that even children can use them without concern. A study published in 2000 demonstrated nice LDL lowering in kids, especially those with particularly high cholesterol levels. There were no side effects.

The only apparent exception to this rule are people born with hypersitosterolemia, a rare metabolic disorder. They absorb phytosterols as readily as cholesterol. But such people are identified by the age of 10. For the rest of us, phytosterols are completely and totally safe.

The Food and Drug Administration has also approved sales of the margarines containing the sterols and stanols as safe and effective. In fact, the FDA gave manufacturers permission in 2000 to state that the plant substances reduce cholesterol and cut the risk of developing coronary heart disease. The FDA rarely allows such health claims. Oats were the first food to obtain such permission.

ANOTHER HEALTH BENEFIT

As they age, many men develop a condition known as benign prostatic hypertrophy (BPH). This means a growth in the size of the prostate gland not associated necessarily with prostate cancer. Such growth puts pressure on the urethra and leads to problems with urination, often causing afflicted men to urinate frequently throughout the day and night.

It turns out that phytosterols are an effective treatment for BPH. A paper published in the June 1995 issue of *The Lancet* revealed that even small amounts of phytosterols (20 mg three times daily for six months) resulted in shrinkage of the prostate gland and reduction of symptoms.

HOW TO USE PHYTOSTEROLS

Both the sterol- and stanol-containing margarines made by Benecol and Take Control will give you an additional LDL reduction when used regularly. It doesn't take much. Just 1 tablespoon of Take Control margarine contains 1250 mg of soybean phytosterols, enough to achieve a nice cholesterol reduction. But you may not want to have margarine with, say, cold cereal in the morning or a low-fat hot dog for lunch. And the margarine may not be available at the restaurant you're eating in. Then there are long weekends and vacations away from home.

A tablet or two of phytosterol prior to meals is the most convenient source. If you take the phytosterols before a meal, the plant sterols get to the micelle receptor sites first, beating cholesterol to the punch.

But what about the 30-minute waiting period? The latest generation of phytosterol tablets produced by Endurance Products and introduced in 2000 provide immediate release. Just swallow one or two tablets at the beginning of meals. Nothing could be more simple.

As with my niacin, I keep a supply of my phytosterol tablets everywhere. I take one 400-mg tablet at the start of each meal, two if I'm having eggs, shrimp, or other food that is particularly rich in cholesterol.

I get my phytosterols every day, without the extra fat, calories, or expense of either brand of margarine. Benecol has introduced gel caps as their alternative, but the price is more than twice that of the Endurance phytosterols. Because Endurance does no advertising and there are no retail store markups, the price is low. And the quality is high.

Endurance phytosterol information can be obtained at 800-483-2532 or www.endur.com. Or write to:

Endurance Products Company
PO Box 230489
Tigard, Oregon 97281-0489

A chewable phytosterol tablet called Kholesterol Blocker is made by Nutrition For Life International. Unfortunately, the chewable convenience comes with a high price. The best I could do is a 10 percent discount for those giving the ID number 152097 when placing an order at 800-800-7377.

Table 7. CHOLESTEROL AND FAT CONTENT OF COMMON FOODS

	Cholesterol (mg)	Fat (g)
Cheese (1 oz)		
American	27	9
Brie	29	8
Cheddar	30	9
Eggs		
One large chicken egg	220	5
Caviar (1 tbsp/40 g)	94	2.9
Fast Foods		
Big Mac	83	35
Wendy's Double Hamburger	150	30
Egg McMuffin (w/ cheese)	260	16
Meats (3.5 oz, cooked)		
Beef brisket, fat and lean	92	35
Round steak	96	15
Tenderloin, fat and lean	86	17
Tenderloin, lean only	84	9
Poultry		
Chicken, dark w/skin	92	16
Chicken, dark wo/skin	93	10
Chicken, light w/skin	84	11
Chicken, light wo/skin	85	4.5
Turkey, dark w/skin	89	11.5
Turkey, dark wo/skin	85	7.2
Turkey, light w/skin	76	8.3
Turkey, light wo/skin	69	3.2
Chicken liver	631	15.5
Shellfish (3.5 oz, raw)		
Clams	29	0.7
Crab	35	0.5
Crayfish	118	0.9
Lobster	81	0.8
Scallops	28	0.6
Shrimp	130	0.6

	Cholesterol (mg)	Fat (g)
Variety Meats (3.5 oz, cooked)		
Brains	2000–2500	10–16
Heart	193	5.6
Kidneys	387	3.4
Liver	389	4.9
Paté (1 oz)	43	5–12
Tripe	95	4.0

8
Niacin:
Fighting for Your Healthy Heart

If asked what is the most important component of my heart protection regimen, there would be no doubt in my mind. Although each and every part of my program plays a vital role, the MVP, the most valuable player, remains the vitamin niacin. I have taken niacin since 1984, never missing a single day. This deceptively simple miracle of nature has done more than anything else to save my life.

When I wrote about niacin in the first edition of this book, I got my share of criticism. Today there is widespread enthusiasm for niacin throughout the medical community. One leading clinical research physician called niacin his "secret weapon against heart disease" at a meeting of the American Heart Association. The National Cholesterol Education Program puts niacin at the top of its list of choices when diet alone isn't enough to bring cholesterol down to normal levels. The medical literature abounds with studies demonstrating the safety and effectiveness of niacin.

Let's start with the fact that 80 percent of all the cholesterol in the bloodstream, whether elevated or not, is made by the body, principally in the liver. Diet plays only a secondary role. That's why the vast majority of people fail, as I did, when trying diet alone to control cholesterol levels. Niacin works in the liver to curtail the production of the bad LDL cholesterol. And, as we'll see in the coming pages, it does much more to protect our hearts.

Niacin, also known as nicotinic acid, is sometimes called vitamin B_3. As a vitamin found in a wide variety of foods, niacin has an RDA of only 20 mg to prevent the deficiency state called pellagra. These small amounts of niacin present in the diet have no effect on cholesterol, but when used in what are termed "pharmacologic doses," niacin battles cholesterol as well as or better than any prescription drug. In fact, doctors writing in the medical journals refer to niacin as a drug because of its dramatic effect on the body.

When niacin enters the bloodstream, the liver proceeds to break it down first to a derivative called niacinamide and finally to nicotinuric acid, which is excreted in the urine. It is during this metabolic process that niacin appears to work its magic.

There in the liver niacin interferes in some way that is not yet fully understood with the formation of very-low-density lipoprotein (VLDL) cholesterol, which is needed to make LDL, low-density lipoprotein cholesterol.

Total and LDL cholesterol levels fall by an average of 20 to 40 percent. This effect has been documented again and again at the University of California, the University of Southern California, the University of Minnesota, the University of North Carolina, and research institutions across the nation and around the world. Today there are literally hundreds of papers published in the most prestigious journals showing niacin's safety and effectiveness.

If niacin were to be introduced today by a major pharmaceutical manufacturer, it would quickly be one of the top prescriptions drugs, making the company millions of dollars. No prescription drug in existence today can come anywhere near niacin in controlling a vast number of CHD risk factors.

In addition to lowering LDL, niacin raises levels of the protective HDL cholesterol. One study at Duke University Medical Center found it more effective than the prescription drug gemfibrozil. That's especially significant when you look at the multicenter investigation that showed how gemfibrozil (usually marketed as Lopid) produced a significant reduction in risk of major cardiovascular events in patients with a previously low HDL count. That particular study was a medical landmark, since it showed how raising low levels of HDL protected against heart disease even when LDL numbers are in the normal range. But why take an expensive prescription drug when inexpensive, over-the-counter niacin does an even better job?

Often HDL improvements can be achieved even with low niacin doses, as documented by physicians at Hadassah University Hospital in Israel. They used less than 500 mg to produce significant HDL gains. At the Mayo Clinic in Rochester, Minnesota, 63 participants in a cardiac rehabilitation program who had low HDL levels experienced an average 18 percent increase with niacin. And doctors at the Ochsner Clinic in New Orleans achieved a 32 percent HDL improvement.

Levels of the blood fat triglycerides fall dramatically with niacin, far more so than with prescribed drugs. The higher the triglyceride problem is to begin with, the more effective niacin is. Patients participating in the Coronary Drug Project, a long-term, nationwide, double-blind study, experienced anywhere from 15 to 30 percent triglyceride reductions. In an NIH-sponsored study, triglycerides fell an average of 52 percent. Regardless of percentage of improvement, niacin can bring triglycerides down to normal even if beginning levels are very high.

The independent risk factor Lp(a) also succombs to niacin, even though it responds to neither diet nor drugs. Lp(a) levels were down 35 percent when subjects were given niacin at the Oregon Health Sciences University. At the internationally renowned Karolinska Institute in Sweden, Lp(a) came down an average of 33 percent in all patients treated with niacin. The Clinical Center of the National Institutes of Health (NIH) reported in the *Journal of the American Medical Association* that "strong consideration should be given to including nicotinic acid as part of the pharmacologic regimen" for treating Lp(a) elevations. NIH cited a potential 50 percent Lp(a) reduction.

Once something that few doctors even knew about, Lp(a) is now recognized as a risk factor that can exert its own deadly influence even when more commonly considered blood fats are more or less normal. Anyone with a strong family history of CHD should be aware of his or her levels.

And niacin exerts its protective influence on even less well known risk factors:

- Small, dense LDL particles are transformed to larger, less dense particles with niacin. Research at the University of California found that those with the smallest particles are at three times the risk as those with the largest LDL particles. And in another study at the same center, niacin was found to significantly increase LDL diameter.
- We know that heart attacks are frequently precipitated by the formation of a blood clot that blocks blood flow to the heart. A number of factors influence the likelihood of clots forming. Fibrinogen is one of those factors and, as such, is considered to be an independent CHD risk factor. Those with high levels of fibrinogen are at significantly greater risk. But fortunately, niacin has the unique characteristic of reducing levels of fibrinogen. No cholesterol-lowering prescription drug has that capacity.
- One of the hot topics at the 2000 AHA annual scientific sessions was the role of platelet aggregation. Platelets are the cells

in the body that begin the clotting process. When particularly "sticky" platelets gather together (aggregate), the likelihood of clotting goes up.

One method the body uses to control platelet aggregation is the balance between two hormone-like substances called prostaglandins. One prostaglandin, termed thromboxane, increases aggregation, while another, prostacyclin, decreases the tendency of platelets to gather. Ideally we would like to tip the balance in favor of prostacyclin, to limit the clotting potential. Niacin does just that.

■ But the bottom line in protection against heart disease remains protection of life itself. The risk of dying of heart attack dropped significantly in patients taking niacin. Those taking niacin as part of the Coronary Drug Project, the longest running such study, were far less likely to suffer a myocardial infarction. Which of niacin's many beneficial effects was responsible? Probably a combination of all. And no prescription drug can match niacin's total performance.

What if your doctor has prescribed one of the statin drugs such as Pravachol or Lipitor? When it comes to reduction of total and LDL cholesterol, no doubt the statins work very well, often even better than niacin. But they do not provide niacin's additional benefits. That's why authorities are using niacin in combination with the statins more and more.

A stellar example of the effectiveness of that combination was reported at the 2000 AHA meeting by doctors from the University of Washington. They gave 160 patients both immediate-release niacin (2 to 4 grams) and the statin drug Zocor (simvastatin) (10 to 20 mg) for three years and then measured arterial blockage with angiograms. Frankly, researchers normally couch their findings in rather cautious scientific terminology. This time they came right to the point in their conclusions that "niacin plus simvastatin have strikingly favorable effects. Atherosclerosis progression is virtually halted and clinical events are reduced by 70 percent with this well-tolerated regimen." Wow! What better testimony could anyone ask for?

That's just one of many studies showing how niacin can boost the effectiveness of statins. The combination is coming into such favor, in fact, that at least one pharmaceutical company will launch a formulation combining niacin and the statin drug lovastatin (marketed as Mevacor). Tested at the Long Beach Veterans Administration Medical Center in California with 814 patients, the drug termed Nicostatin increased HDL levels 30 percent in the first four months and 41 percent at the end of a year. LDL levels dropped 45 percent, triglycerides fell by 42 percent, and Lp(a) came down by 18 percent.

While that is of course a glowing testament to the niacin-statin combination, many question the concept of a fixed combination. Depending on the particular patient's case, dosage of either the niacin or the statin may vary.

If you currently take a statin drug prescribed by your doctor, please discuss the possibility of such a combination with him or her. Even though your LDL may be controlled by the statin, the niacin can provide additional benefit for HDL, triglycerides, Lp(a), fibrinogen, small, dense LDL, and prostaglandin balance. Such a chat with your doctor could literally save your life.

Why don't doctors recommend niacin more often? Since niacin is a relatively inexpensive vitamin supplement, available at any pharmacy, health food store, or through mail order, manufacturers do not send sales representatives into doctors' offices. Conversely, pharmaceutical companies enjoy huge profits from drug sales and deluge physicians with information about their products.

Moreover, statin drugs are easier for doctors to work with than niacin. Most do not want to spend the time counseling patients about how to take niacin, preferring the convenience of simply writing a prescription for a statin drug.

According to one of niacin's pioneering researchers, Dr. William Parsons of Scottsdale, Arizona, "If every doctor in the country were good at niacin and would use it in preference to other medications, probably 90 percent or more of patients needing cholesterol control could take it successfully. This would literally save billions every year." Not to speak of saving many, many lives.

Is niacin a vitamin or a drug? In medical jargon, doctors and researchers refer to niacin in large doses as a drug. They use that term because in those large pharmacologic doses, niacin has an effect on the body beyond its role as a vitamin preventing pellagra. In that respect, researchers also call large doses of vitamin C—or any supplement—a drug.

Certainly niacin should be used with respect and caution. As I will detail in the coming pages, large doses of niacin have the potential for certain adverse reactions or side effects. Since it works in the liver to correct cholesterol problems, and it is metabolized there, niacin does place a certain extra load on that organ. As a result, those taking it should see their doctors regularly to have their liver functions checked. And because niacin does have a number of contraindications, not everyone should take it. Everyone should discuss niacin with his or her physician before starting treatment.

NIACIN'S SIDE EFFECTS, ADVERSE EFFECTS, AND CONTRAINDICATIONS

Virtually everyone taking standard, unmodified, crystalline niacin experiences the "niacin flush." Some people react more strongly than others. While the reaction is totally harmless, it can be uncomfortable. Some describe the flush as a reddening of the skin along with a prickly, burning sensation; it occurs 20 to 30 minutes after taking a dose of niacin and lasts 10 to 20 minutes on average. Flushing typically diminishes as one continues to take niacin and the body becomes accustomed to it.

With time-release or sustained-release niacin, the flush can occur as long as 2 hours after the dosage. For practically everyone, this is a tiny price to pay for the benefits being derived. Even after 17 years of niacin, I still get some flushing now and then, though much less than at first. Whenever I feel the flush I think of how the niacin is acting to lower my cholesterol and risk of heart disease. I view it in a very positive way. So should you.

One can lessen the niacin flush in a number of ways. First, it's best to take niacin with food, at mealtime, and with plenty of fluids. Second, taking an aspirin tablet prior to the niacin eliminates or at least weakens the flush. Third, one can take modified niacin in slow-release formulations. One such preparation, which I will discuss more fully, practically wipes out the niacin flush.

Some may experience a variety of gastrointestinal disturbances with niacin. I've found that to be the case mostly in those who take certain slow-release formulations, which include other ingredients to slow down the niacin's release. It appears to be those other agents, known as "excipients," that present the problems. However, any niacin tablet or capsule can produce gastrointestinal upset occasionally. Not often, but it does happen.

Many niacin users report itching to one degree or another. Dry skin occasionally accompanies its use. In rare instances, one may develop a rash, typically on the chest and shoulders. Such a rash indicates an inability to tolerate niacin and it should be discontinued.

Niacin lowers glucose tolerance, the body's ability to maintain fairly constant blood sugar levels, to a certain extent. This is not a problem for normal, healthy individuals but may be a consideration for diabetics, who must monitor their blood sugar closely.

In the past, doctors thought niacin was off-limits to their diabetic patients. But doctors from a number of centers, reporting in the September 2000 issue of the *Journal of the American Medical Association,* concluded that based on their work with 125 diabetic patients, niacin is both safe and highly effective in this group. While glucose levels were modestly increased by niacin, the impact was not significant. Moreover, levels of the more important HbA 1c (hemoglobin A1c) were unchanged. That factor is the state-of-the-art approach to physicians' monitoring of glucose tolerance.

That's really good news for diabetic patients, since the disease is associated with much more risk for heart disease. Those receiving niacin saw HDL levels climb 29 percent, triglycerides fall by 23 percent, and LDL levels drop 8 percent. That greatly reduces CHD risk.

Development of a vision problem termed "maculopathy" has been reported to occur in approximately 0.67 percent of patients taking niacin. The condition is completely reversible when one stops treatment. The authors of a report on niacin-induced maculopathy stated that "only those who experience visual symptoms need to be ophthalmologically evaluated." This is truly rare and has been associated with doses higher than most authorities feel are needed for cholesterol control—definitely higher than what I personally use and recommend. Check with your doctor if you do happen to develop blurred vision; if niacin is responsible, your physician will either modify your dosage or suggest that you discontinue use.

Niacin may slightly increase the production of uric acid in the blood. For the vast majority of people, this poses no problem, since uric acid levels remain comfortably within normal limits. However, even slight elevations of uric acid can result in episodes of gout in those who have that disorder to begin with.

Most important, doctors should routinely monitor liver function by testing for liver enzymes in the blood of those taking niacin. Slight elevations in those enzymes are not cause for alarm and are rather common in niacin takers.

Dr. Robert Kreisberg of the University of Alabama School of Medicine put the matter of niacin and liver function into a clear perspective in an editorial in the October 1994 issue of the *American Journal of Medicine.* He wrote:

> Increased liver enzymes become an indication for stopping niacin therapy only when they are more than three times the

upper-normal limit. In my experience, I have found that physicians are too quick to discontinue niacin, and for that matter, other hypolipidemic drugs (the statin cholesterol-lowering drugs) because of mild or trivial changes in liver enzymes and explain to patients that the drug was 'hurting their liver'; perhaps this is understandable in our litigious society.

In practical terms, how many people will be able to take niacin? The issue of flushing is really a matter of nuisance. Unpleasant for some, sure, but such flushing tends to dissipate quickly after one's body gets used to the niacin. Increases in uric acid and decreases in glucose tolerance are not significant for the vast majority. Gastrointestinal disturbances can be eliminated by switching brands. A Mayo Clinic study found that all participants were able to take niacin without intolerable side effects.

How often should one check liver enzymes? After your doctor approves niacin for you, he or she will want to test your liver enzymes in about two to three months. If all's well, as it most likely will be, the next test should be six months later. Most physicians will want to run liver enzyme tests twice a year thereafter, right along with your cholesterol test, done with the same blood sample.

CONTRAINDICATIONS TO NIACIN USE

Some people should not take niacin at all. The contraindications to niacin use include pregnancy, severe cardiac arrhythmias, active peptic ulcer, gout, and prior liver disorders including hepatitis and cirrhosis. Other contraindications may be a previous inability to tolerate niacin as shown by severe skin rash or greatly elevated liver enzymes if those conditions did not respond to dosage modifications, and heavy alcohol use or abuse with possible subclinical liver damage that would not normally be detected until the liver is further challenged by niacin.

Why bother to take niacin when there are so many possible side effects and adverse reactions? Well, first of all, I don't think everyone should take it. Of all the men and women whose lipids need modification, many will be able to slash their risks by employing the other aspects of the program in this book. Dietary modifications, soluble fibers, and phytosterols can and will dramatically help many cholesterol problems and will greatly reduce CHD risk, especially when combined with regular exercise, stress reduction and relaxation techniques, and supplements such as folic acid to control risk factors such as homocysteine.

Second, virtually all substances have the potential for adverse reactions. Millions of men and women take aspirin daily. Yet the list of side effects and adverse reactions is so long that many would be frightened away if they ever saw it. The same goes for many over-the-counter drugs. I list all these considerations not only out of a feeling that my readers deserve full disclosure, but also since bottles of niacin do not state them.

Third, niacin truly can be a lifesaver for millions of people. As one who has come to the precipice of death, I view heart disease as a personal enemy. There is no way for me to express my strong emotions when I think of those who needlessly suffer heart attacks and die because of coronary heart disease. I am firmly convinced that niacin has helped to save my life and that it just might save yours.

Fourth, when is one truly safe? Many physicians are pleased when their patients' cholesterol levels fall to 200 or so, even though HDLs remain low and triglycerides are elevated. That's true even for some taking statin drugs. *Such men and women are at continued risk!* Heart disease is largely preventable, but that means getting total cholesterol down into the 150 to 160 range (no higher than 180), with triglycerides down well under 150, and HDL over 40 for men and 45 for women. Niacin can help make that happen, as well as dealing with the other risk factors I've identified in this chapter.

WHAT IF I CAN'T TAKE NIACIN?

For a small percentage of men and women, niacin is definitely contraindicated. While I believe that niacin should be the first choice, if that is not possible one must consider alternatives. If lifestyle modifications and other supplements do not adequately control your cholesterol levels, talk with your doctor about a prescription for one of the statin drugs. The safety of the statins has been well established in the millions of patients who have used them since the first such agent, Mevacor (lovastatin), was approved in 1987. The importance of controlling the full lipid profile is so great that I think one should do whatever is necessary to eliminate those risks. And of course, if you and your doctor decide on a prescription drug, simply use it to replace the niacin in this complete program. By doing so you will ensure maximum impact on risk.

Not all statins are created equal. Some are more potent than others. Zocor appears to reduce LDL more dramatically than Pravachol, and Lipitor is the most potent of them all, with better effects on HDL and triglycerides as well.

Even for those unable to take niacin as a first-line defense against cholesterol, it might be possible to combine a low dosage along with a statin drug to provide the additional benefits from niacin. Don't fail to discuss that possibility with your doctor.

HOW TO TAKE NIACIN

As I have said, before taking niacin, be sure to discuss it with your physician. He or she may have suggestions regarding appropriate dosages. I provide the following information as reference for both you and your doctor. In fact, you may wish to bring this chapter to his or her attention.

To achieve cholesterol reductions, doses of niacin have ranged up to 8 grams of the immediate-release formulation a day and more. However, much lower doses have been shown to be effective, especially in combination with other approaches.

The maximum daily niacin dose should not exceed 3000 mg (3 grams) of standard, crystalline, immediate-release (IR) niacin or 1500 mg (1.5 grams) of slow-release or sustained-release (SR) niacin. SR niacin formulations have been noted to have both twice the effectiveness and twice the toxicity of IR preparations, hence the difference in maximum dosages. Those dosages have been shown to provide maximum benefits while resulting in minimal side effects. Larger doses are more likely to result in adverse reactions, including abnormal liver enzymes.

For those with exceptionally high total and LDL cholesterol levels, it is better to consider a combination of niacin and a prescription drug rather than trying to increase niacin dosages.

When used exclusively for the purpose of raising abnormally low levels of the protective HDL cholesterol, lower dosages are often effective. Research in Israel has indicated that a daily dose of 500 mg of IR niacin can significantly raise HDLs, while also lowering triglycerides somewhat.

To be most effective, niacin doses should be divided and taken three times daily, preferably with meals. While twice-a-day or even once-daily dosing may be more convenient, it is not as effective. That includes even the new prescription-only niacin formulation, Niaspan.

To be sure I don't forget to take my niacin, I keep a supply in my bathroom, kitchen, car, office, attaché case, golf bag, and travel toiletry kit. I use divided containers found in all pharmacies to store both the niacin and other supplements for the week. Carrying it along becomes a habit one thinks about no more than any other. And this is a good habit.

Traditionally, niacin therapy is begun at low doses and is gradually increased to minimize the flush and to allow the body to become accustomed to it. While your physician may have other recommendations, which you should follow, the following dosage schedule for initiating niacin therapy has been suggested frequently in the medical literature to achieve a final dosage of 3000 mg of IR niacin:

First three days	One 100-mg tablet three times daily = 300 mg
Next three days	Two 100-mg tablets three times daily = 600 mg
Next three days	Three 100-mg tablets three times daily = 900 mg
Next three days	Four 100-mg tablets three times daily = 1200 mg
Next three days	One 500 mg tablet three times daily = 1500 mg
Next three days	One 100-mg tablet plus one 500-mg tablet 3 times daily = 1800 mg
Next three days	Two 100-mg tablets plus one 500-mg tablet 3 times daily = 2100 mg
Next three days	Three 100-mg tablets plus one 500-mg tablet 3 times daily = 2400 mg
Next three days	Four 100-mg tablets plus one 500-mg tablet 3 times daily = 2700 mg
From then on	Two 500-mg tablets three times daily = 3000 mg

SR NIACIN TO REDUCE FLUSH

Companies use a variety of formulations to produce an SR niacin that reduces or even eliminates flush. Some are simply compressed more tightly to slow down the dissolution process. Others add ingredients to create a more gradual release into the blood. One patented product, Endur-acin, uses a unique wax matrix to release a given amount of niacin at first, and then a gradual trickle over a number of hours.

Beginning in 1990 a number of reports warned against the potential hazards of SR niacin. Concerns were based on a case history involving a man who at his physician's prescription had been taking a daily dose of 6000 mg (6 grams) of IR niacin. He then switched to an SR niacin formulation he purchased at a health food store. By doing so, the man effectively and inadvertently doubled his dosage to 12,000 mg (12 grams) of niacin daily. The result was tragic—liver failure and the need for a liver transplant.

That, of course, was an extreme case. Nothing like that ever happened again. But subsequent studies did indeed show the increased toxicity of SR niacin. The results show that a given dose of SR niacin is the equivalent of twice the dose of IR niacin.

The SR niacin, per se, was not responsible in the case cited above. The dosage was extreme. Moreover, the man should have had his liver enzymes checked regularly; elevations would have signaled a problem well in advance of any damage. But many stores—and authorities—overreacted and discontinued sales of SR niacin. Reports urged that SR formulations be banned and only IR be sold.

SR niacin is completely safe when taken properly and monitored by a physician. I began taking niacin in 1984 to control my own cholesterol levels. At that time, and for the next four years, I took 3 grams of IR niacin daily. My liver enzymes were always monitored and remained in the normal zone. The flush didn't bother me too much.

Then in 1998 I learned about Endur-acin, a newly developed SR niacin. The maximum dosage is 1500 mg, and it was said to be free of nuisance flushing and gastrointestinal upset. So I tried it. Sure enough, the flush disappeared and my cholesterol levels were actually better than before. I've used Endur-acin ever since.

This is one of the few SR niacin preparations to be clinically evaluated. A study done at the University of Minnesota found Endur-acin to be safe and effective. The dropout rate was only 3.4 percent, and participants had no problem in complying with the niacin dosage of one 500-mg tablet three times daily.

The investigator, Dr. Joseph Keenan, also reported that doses of 2000 mg a day resulted in elevated liver enzymes with no further improvements in cholesterol values.

As an interesting side note, some individuals have noticed that the Endur-acin tablet appears occasionally in the bowel movement and worried that the niacin was passing through the system unabsorbed. Actually the niacin is leached from the wax matrix tablet and by the time it may appear in the stool, all the niacin is removed.

A sample dosage schedule for SR niacin may be as follows:

First week	One 250-mg tablet morning and evening = 500 mg
Second week	One 250-mg tablet morning, noon, and evening = 750 mg
Third week	Two 250-mg tablets or one 500-mg three times daily = 1500 mg
Thereafter	One 500-mg tablet morning, noon, and evening = 1500 mg

COMBINATION IR AND SR NIACIN REGIMEN

Through the years I've continued to monitor the medical literature regarding niacin and its benefits for cholesterol control and prevention of heart disease. From a report in early 1994, I learned that researchers had found that SR niacin lowered LDL cholesterol significantly more than IR niacin did. Conversely, IR niacin did a better job of increasing HDL and lowering triglycerides.

That led to the next stage of self-experimentation with niacin. I came up with a combination of SR and IR niacin formulations to achieve the best of both worlds. For me, and subsequently for others, it is the best approach for controlling LDL, HDL, and triglycerides.

Morning   One 500-mg SR niacin (Endur-acin) plus one 500-mg IR niacin
Afternoon One 500-mg IR niacin
Evening   One 500-mg SR niacin (Endur-acin)

Note that I have substituted my previous afternoon dosage of one 500-mg SR niacin (Endur-acin) with two 500-mg IR niacin tablets, which I take in the morning and afternoon. Remember that 500 mg of SR equals 1000 mg of IR. Therefore, the effective total dosage remains the same.

BUT THOSE NIACIN SUBSTITUTES DON'T WORK!

Virtually every medical report on the subject begins with words to the effect that "niacin is an effective treatment for lowering cholesterol." Fortunately, as an over-the-counter supplement, niacin remains very inexpensive, especially compared with prescription drugs. But be cautious about choosing among the niacin preparations you see for sale. Not all of them work.

Niacinamide is the metabolic breakdown product of niacin. Used in supplements, it satisfies one's vitamin requirement for niacin. But it has no effect on lowering cholesterol.

Inositol nicotinate is sometimes labeled a "no-flush" niacin, but like niacinamide, it doesn't lower cholesterol regardless of claims made on the bottle or by salespersons in health stores. There is no clinical evidence that inositol nicotinate has any effect on cholesterol. It may also be labeled as inositol hexanicotinate.

You might also see combination niacin products on the shelves. These products may also include dietary fibers, antioxidants, and other supplements. The amounts of niacin are typically too low to have an effect on cholesterol. If a combination includes, let's say, 50 mg of niacin, you would have to take a lot of those capsules or tablets to reach an effective dosage. Avoid those combinations, as they just don't work.

NIACIN IN PERSPECTIVE

My recommendations on niacin were frequently criticized when my book was first published. Some uninformed individuals said it didn't work. Others felt such advice should only come from physicians. There is no point in my responding to past criticism. I am glad I got the word out regarding this potential lifesaver.

Today niacin is far better understood, recognized, and prescribed by doctors. They, and now you, know about its unparalleled and unequaled benefits in the fight against heart disease.

9
What's Hot, What's Not

As we learn more and more about heart disease and its causes, we also discover ways of preventing CHD. This book is filled with information and focuses on the best approaches you and I can take to protect our hearts. In some cases, a particular type of intervention is so important that I've devoted entire chapters. The uses of niacin and soluble fibers are examples.

In this chapter I turn to less well established modalities. Some are potent alternatives or may add just the little boost your own particular regimen might need. Others provide tantalizing ideas future research may or may not confirm as valuable. And, sadly, a few are not only absolutely worthless, but they represent money-making schemes by those who would take advantage of people desperate for help.

Let's start on a positive note with one of my personal favorites.

SEX AND CHD RISK

According to a British cardiologist who had done his research with 2400 men in Wales, having sex three or four times a week reduces the risk of heart attack or stroke by half. At the start of the study, the men were asked whether they had sex once, twice, or three or more times a week. During follow-up in the next ten years, men who reported having orgasms three or more times weekly were half as likely to have had a heart attack or stroke.

Why is sex protective? There are several possible reasons. First, of course, it's relaxing and enjoyable. Second, especially for older individuals, frequent sexual activity may reflect excellent physical health. Third, regular sex is more likely when one's emotions are under control; conversely, sexual activity is likely to decrease when one is under a lot of stress or is depressed. Fourth, perhaps sexual activity contributes to one's total exercise for the week. Maybe there is a wonderful link we haven't discovered yet but frequent sexual activity may simply be a marker of a generally healthy lifestyle.

While we're on this subject, it's worth noting that Viagra has been shown to be completely safe, even for those with diagnosed heart disease. The only contraindications would be current use of prescribed nitrate drugs.

ASPIRIN AND YOUR HEART

While not as much fun, a daily aspirin tablet provides enormous protection against heart attack. Its principal mode of action makes platelets in the blood less sticky and therefore less likely to form clots. Aspirin also appears to have a protective effect on the endothelial lining of the arteries. And it may reduce inflammation in the heart in much the same way it does with arthritis.

Certainly every man and woman (we have well-established data for both genders) with either diagnosed heart disease or existing risk factors such as hypertension should take aspirin. Many doctors believe that almost everyone would derive potential benefit with very little risk. Ask your own physician.

Medical consensus calls for one 81-mg aspirin tablet daily, with a "booster" of one 325-mg tablet twice a month. Some think those who can tolerate it without gastric upset might benefit from a daily 325-mg dose.

How much benefit are we talking about here? Daily aspirin use may reduce the incidence of nonfatal heart attack by more than 30 percent in people at high risk. Data also indicate that aspirin may also help prevent heart attack in men over age 50 even if they do not fit into the high-risk category.

Not only can aspirin help prevent heart attack, it is the first line of treatment for anyone suffering an MI. Chew one 325-mg tablet if you think you might be having a heart attack. That gets the aspirin into the bloodstream faster than swallowing with water. Taken at the first symptom, aspirin can help to break up a clot that is limiting blood flow to the heart's muscle.

ARGININE AND ENDOTHELIAL HEALTH

Several years ago researchers determined that some unknown substance kept arteries flexible and healthy. They only knew that it originated in the lining of the arteries, and so they termed the mystery chemical EDRF, for endothelium-derived relaxation factor.

Eventually they learned that EDRF was actually nitric oxide (NO), an agent that was formed and then broken down so quickly and in such minute quantities that it had previously escaped detection.

Those producing more NO had healthier arteries. The endothelium was more elastic and able to dilate, allowing for greater blood flow when needed.

To make NO the body needs a supply of the amino acid arginine. In fact, recent investigations have shown tremendous endothelial improvement in those getting large quantities of arginine, doses up to 8 grams (8000 mg).

So how might one get the amino acid? A product called the Heart Bar supplies 6 grams in two bars, the recommended daily intake by the manufacturers. But the bars are expensive, and don't taste particularly good, and you are not likely to eat them day in and day out.

What about getting arginine from food? The typical U.S. diet provides 5 grams of arginine or less daily. Some foods are far better sources than others. One cup of low-fat cottage cheese packs about 1200 mg. An ounce of cheddar or other cheeses contains around 250 mg. One large egg has just short of 400 mg, half from the white and half from the yolk. A 3-ounce serving of fish provides about 1000 mg; most people eat twice that much. Look to red meats for a lot of arginine, with an average of more than 1500 mg per 3.5-ounce serving. The arginine in nuts may be what helps protect the heart health of those who regularly snack on them. One ounce of peanuts packs nearly 1000 mg, the same for 2 tabespoons of peanut butter. Other plant foods do not have much arginine.

You can also find arginine supplements in any health food store. Tablets typically contain 500 mg. Between food and supplements, you should have no problem getting several grams of arginine daily.

Since I began this chapter with the joyous news that sex is good for you, it is worth noting that Viagra, which sells for several dollars a tablet and most insurance plans don't cover it, works by increasing production of NO, just like arginine. How's that for some bonus points?

CARNITINE FOR CLAUDICATION

Carnitine is another amino acid. Researchers in Italy have found that supplements provide a lot of benefit for those suffering from intermittent claudication, the medical term for severe cramping pain in the legs due to insufficient blood flow through clogged arteries in the lower limbs. Those with the worst cases improved most, improving their ability to walk greater distances without pain.

But there's a fly in the ointment. The only form of the amino acid that works is proprionyl-L-carnitine, which is available only in Europe. Carnitine supplements in U.S. health food stores don't do the trick. Hopefully the FDA will give its approval to the effective form so that it can become available in the United States as well.

ANOTHER KIND OF VITAMIN E

Tocotrienols are the chemical cousins of the more familiar vitamin E, tocopherol. Tocotrienols benefit the heart in three separate but important ways. First, they are even more potent antioxidants than their tocopherol counterparts, preventing the oxidation of LDL and Lp(a) cholesterol. Ideally, one would take both forms of vitamin E. Second, tocotrienols provide a small but significant lowering of LDL, as well as Lp(a). Third, users will enjoy protection of the endothial lining of the heart's arteries. It appears that tocotrienols limit arterial damage and help keep arteries more elastic and flexible.

The first research on tocotrienols was done with barley-derived materials. Today tocotrienols are manufactured from either rice bran oil or palm oil. Interestingly, both those oils were shown to have a cholesterol-lowering effect before it was known that they were rich in tocotrienols prior to filtering. While neither oil is common in the United States, one can easily find tocotrienol supplements.

Evolve, produced from rice bran oil, is currently available only by direct order from the company at 800-508-7432. Care-Diem is a blend of tocotrienols, found in health food stores and pharmacies. Two companies in Malaysia, Golden Hope and Hovid, make tocotrienols from palm oil; their products are also sold here in the United States.

EFFECTIVE CHOLESTEROL LOWERING

I've been a fan, advocate, and user of niacin since 1984, as the best approach to cholesterol reduction and protection against other CHD risk factors. But there are definitely other agents that work to control artery-clogging lipids.

Statin Drugs

The imposing designation for these prescription-only cholesterol-lowering drugs is "HMG co-A reductase inhibitors." The first, lovastatin (Mevacor) got FDA approval in 1987. Since that time, several statin drugs have been developed and approved for use in the United States and internationally. They all work by inhibiting the liver's production of a particular enzyme necessary for the body's manufacture of cholesterol. Some are more potent than others. Simvastatin (Zocor) is more powerful than lovastatin (Mevacor), and atorvastatin (Lipitor) is the most potent of them all.

Early concerns over potential side effects including cataract development were apparently not warranted. Muscular aching, termed rhabdomyolysis, which can lead to permanent deterioration of muscle tissue, is infrequent but should be reported to your physician immediately. Those taking the statin drugs should have liver enzymes checked on a regular basis, typically every six months or so. That's also the case for niacin, which also works in the liver. And there have been reports of loss of sexual libido with the statins.

All that said, however, the potential side effects do not come close to canceling out the tremendous benefit potential. A very effective way to lower cholesterol, the statin drugs have been proven to prevent heart attacks and save lives. They are extremely easy to take: Typical dosage is one tiny tablet at bedtime.

Statin drug takers should be aware of a little known food-drug interaction involving grapefruit. Several studies have all come to the same conclusion. Grapefruit vastly increases the amount of statins in the blood—by as much as 12-fold. Although grapefruit is an excellent food and source of vitamin C, statin users should probably avoid it.

If diet fails to lower cholesterol levels sufficiently, or if a patient has an extremely high cholesterol level to begin with that is unlikely to be totally improved by diet alone, most doctors will immediately reach for the prescription pad and write out an order for a statin drug. Again, those drugs are relatively safe and very effective. But I still prefer niacin by a country mile.

No statin can raise HDL, lower triglycerides, slash Lp(a), convert small, dense LDL molecules into safer large, buoyant particles, and decrease the likelihood of blood clots as well as niacin. Doctors in the know first use niacin.

If your doctor is adamant about your using a statin drug, make a copy of the niacin chapter for him or her to read. Even those who wind up using one of the statins would benefit tremendously by taking the drug in combination with niacin. We have solid data demonstrating how that combination can, as the chief investigator put it, "virtually halt the progression of coronary artery disease."

Cholestin: Over-the-Counter Statin

For decades, if not centuries, Chinese herbalists have used the yeast grown on red rice for heart health. And Chinese chefs use the substance to give the typical red color to dishes such as Peking duck. As is the case with many—but not all—herbal therapies, this one really works.

Chemical analysis reveals that red rice yeast yields lovastatin, the active ingredient in Mevacor. This is a lower-potency natural source of the prescription drug. It is marketed as Cholestin and is available in drug and health food stores. You can expect about a 10 percent cholesterol reduction with daily use as directed on the package.

Urged on by the pharmaceutical manufacturers (no surprise), the FDA has tried to stop manufacture and sales of Cholestin. But thus far, the FDA has failed in its efforts to keep it off the market.

The argument is that Cholestin is a statin, and statin is a drug, and drugs should be FDA-regulated and available only by prescription so that doctors can monitor patients. Sounds okay, but remember that Cholestin is a much less potent form of lovastatin. Ironically, Merck, Mevacor's maker, has petitioned the FDA to allow over-the-counter sales of its drug in reduced potency.

If you do decide to add Cholestin to your heart-health regimen, let your doctor know you are taking it. He or she will no doubt want to monitor your liver function, especially if you're combining the Cholestin with niacin. Again, if it's a choice between cholestin or niacin, go with the niacin.

Guggulipid: A Cure from India

Just as the Chinese doctors have used red rice yeast, Ayurvedic physicians in India have relied on a plant-derived substance called guggulipid, sometimes simply called guggul. The active ingredients have been clinically proven to lower cholesterol by reducing the liver's production. A dosage of 50 mg twice daily achieved a 12 percent reduction in LDL and triglycerides in one study with 61 subjects. But research, especially quality research, is scant. There is little doubt, however, that guggulipid is another alternative or perhaps even an addition that could improve your lipid profile.

HERBS AND YOUR HEART

"I'd rather take herbs than use drugs. I prefer things natural." At first glance there is nothing wrong with that opinion. But in reality, there's not much difference between the two in most cases.

Today we have a drug called aspirin. Good for headaches, arthritis, even heart health. Then there is the cure, brewed up by Native Americans way before Columbus from the bark of the willow tree. Both have the active ingredient acetylsalicylic acid.

Again going back in time to Merry Olde England, women healers—often branded witches—gave an extract from the foxglove plant to those with heart ailments. Today doctors prescribe the same agent, digitalis, in tablet form.

The list goes on and on. Many books have been written on traditional native cures. But here's a question for you: if you wouldn't go into a pharmacy and simply pop a digitalis tablet or two without your doctor's supervision, why would you take an herbal agent that might have the same potency and potential adverse reactions?

Many herbs today can provide wonderful alternatives to one problem or another. Indeed, as time goes on we will learn more about valuable herbal remedies and in some cases the active ingredient will be isolated and made into tablets. (Dare I say drugs?) But herbs are not always benign. Like over-the-counter and prescription drugs, they come with potential side effects, adverse reactions, and food and drug interactions. They're not to be treated lightly. Here are some examples to keep in mind:

- *Hawthorne* can block the beneficial effects of medications used for congestive heart failure.
- *St. John's wort* cancels out antirejection drugs given after heart transplants.
- *Ginkgo* multiplies the blood-thinning effects of the prescription drug Coumadin as well as those of aspirin and fish oils.
- *Ma huang* is simply a Chinese herbal source of the drug ephedrine and raises blood pressure and heart rate as much as amphetamines.
- *Ginseng* has an adverse effect on those with hypertension.
- *Aloe* can cause abnormal heart rhythms in pregnant women and children.
- *Black cohosh* can lower blood pressure to dangerous levels.
- *Licorice root* raises blood pressure.

■ *Goldenseal* interferes with blood-thinning drugs and can raise blood pressure.

Need more cause for alarm? Often the workers hired in remote areas of the world to harvest herbs pick the wrong plants, which then become mixed with the desired herbs with toxic results. Many herbs, especially those coming from China, are contaminated with mercury and arsenic.

At this time the FDA has little or no regulatory powers over herbal remedies. It is quite decidedly a situation of "buyer beware." Pharmacies in Germany and elsewhere in Europe provide herbs that are standardized for potency and accuracy in dosage. You have no assurances about herbs sold here in the United States. Personally, I do not use them.

PANTETHINE SHOWS PROMISE

Pantethine is the biologically active form of pantothenic acid, which is a member of the B vitamin complex. At this time, there is no established recommended dietary allowance for the nutrient. Dietary deficiencies are extremely rare, as pantothenic acid is available from a wide variety of foods, including meats, eggs, and dairy. But pantethine, much like niacin, influences lipids in the blood when taken in large doses.

A flurry of research studies in the mid-1980s established that pantethine could reduce total and LDL cholesterol, raise HDL, and lower triglycerides. Additionally, the substance seems to aid in the breakdown of cholesterol by increasing levels of an enzyme called cholesterol esterase.

Unfortunately, for whatever reason, research efforts with pantethine died down, and most of the early investigations were animal studies. But now Japanese researchers have revisited this approach to cholesterol control in a few human studies, all of which show a small but significant degree of improvement in LDL, HDL, and triglycerides.

Although this is very preliminary evidence, and based on only one patient, namely myself, pantethine does indeed show significant promise. I've always had a problem with keeping my HDL up and my triglycerides down. In the past, I've been happy with HDL lab reports in the very low 40s, and with tryglycerides somewhat under 150. But since I have added a 300-mg tablet of pantethine in the morning and another in the evening, for a total of 600 mg daily, my HDL shot up to 48 and my triglycerides dropped down to 86. That's pretty remarkable. Again, this is not solid science, done with many subjects in a closely controlled study. But it sure is a good start. If HDL and triglycerides are concerns for you, give pantethine a try.

Pantothenic acid itself does not, apparently, confer the same benefits. Pantethine is marketed by just a few companies in the United States, although it is widely sold as a prescription drug in Japan, where it is made by Daiichi Pharmaceutical. That company now sells its product here as Pantesin, an over-the-counter dietary supplement. Endurance Products Company now sells bottles of 200 300-mg tablets as Pantethine from Pantesin. Other pantethine products are available in drug and health food stores.

CAN CHITOSAN BLOCK FAT?

You may have seen infomercials for fat blockers under various brand names. The active ingredient, whether in tablets or a solution, is chitosan. Unappetizing as it sounds, chitosan is essentially shells of shrimp and other crustaceans, which are ground into a fine powder and purified.

Television commercials show chitosan mixed into a glass beaker containing water into which oil has been poured. The chitosan binds onto the fat, and large globules drop to the bottom. It looks pretty convincing—and chitosan is indeed used in industry to "mop up" oil in various situations—but does it grab onto and bind fat in your digestive tract from the foods you eat? That's the questionable claim.

Any trained scientist can tell you that what happens in a glass beaker (in vitro) is not necessarily what will happen in the human body (in vivo). Researchers at the University of California at Davis put it to the test.

They used a product called Fat Trapper, which the Federal Trade Commission (FTC) had investigated owing to its claims of weight loss and the ability to block dietary fat. Volunteers were placed on a relatively high-fat diet containing 135 grams of fat daily. Stool samples were collected before and after taking chitosan. Lab analysis found no difference in fecal fat levels. The FTC has ordered the company to "cease and desist" making unsubstantiated claims. The second shoe fell with publication of a study comparing the fat-binding capabilities of chitosan with the prescription-only drug Orlistat. Orlistat is used under a physician's supervision as part of weight-loss programs. Twelve healthy volunteers took one or the other substance for a week, and then for another week switched from one to the other. Those taking Orlistat averaged an additional 16 grams of fat on average in a daily collection of feces, while those receiving chitosan showed no additional fat in the feces. The results were published in the June 2001 issue of the *Journal of Obesity Research*.

The flipside of the story is a small study appearing in the *Journal of the American Nutraceutical Association,* and sponsored by the company that makes the product in question. First, that's not a well-respected journal, and second, there is obvious bias when a company studies its own products. But the data did show that their particular chitosan product did produce significant weight loss without any dietary changes. And there was a small but not statistically significant amount of fat found in the feces of a subgroup of the patients studied.

The chitosan issue is not settled and cast in bronze as of yet. Additional research will supply some missing answers to crucial questions. Does chitosan really block fat in the foods we eat? Does it influence weight loss by way of a mechanism beyond fat blockage? Time will tell. At this time, chitosan must be viewed as ineffective.

CLA: A POTENTIAL WEIGHT-LOSS AID

Conjugated linoleic acid (CLA) is a type of fat found in dairy products, meats, poultry, and eggs. New preliminary findings point to the intriguing notion that CLA in concentrated supplemental form can reduce body fat.

Norwegian researchers reported in the *Journal of Nutrition* in January 2000 that doses of 3.4 grams and 6.8 grams of CLA produced significant body fat reduction over a 12-week period. Animal studies have previously shown similar results.

But this is a new frontier, with a lot of exploring left to be done before I or others make recommendations. You can find CLA in many health food stores. It appears to be safe, but whether it's truly effective remains to be seen.

OUR SUPPLEMENTS ARE SPECIAL!

That's the kind of hype that separates a lot of people from their money. Let's take a simple example. Vitamin C is vitamin C is vitamin C no matter where it comes from, whether oranges or tablets or rose hips. Your body can't tell the difference. So when some infomercial or salesperson tries to tell you that a particular brand is superior, your immediate response should be, "Bunk!"

Companies have made fortunes selling relatively small amounts of minerals dissolved in water. They claim the water comes from glaciers or lakes or streams in parts of the world where people live to ripe old ages. More bunk.

All that said, there can be differences in quality and dosage accuracy. What you read on the label may not always be what you get in the tablets in the bottle. Again, the FDA has little or no regulation over sales of dietary supplements of any kind. Manufacturers and marketers walk a fine line in the claims they make, using words like "promotes heart health" rather than "cures heart disease."

So how do you know what you're getting? One source of reliable information comes from ConsumerLabs.com. That organization regularly tests various supplements and posts the results on their Internet Web site of the same name. And having worked with them for well over a decade, I can personally vouch for the supplements sold by Endurance Products. The quality and formulation are excellent and the prices are reasonable.

"NO-FLUSH" NIACIN PRODUCTS

Probably the biggest reason doctors don't recommend niacin more often is that they have to explain the nuisance side effect of flushing to patients. Indeed, all niacin formulations can produce an uncomfortable burning sensation known as the flush, to one degree or another. And many people, having experienced that flush, aren't willing to put up with it despite the tremendous benefits to be derived.

That's where the unscrupulous marketers come in to prey on the uniformed and unwary individual. They label their products "no flush" niacin, and indeed they produce no flush. Unfortunately they also have no effect on cholesterol levels. That's because those products are not niacin at all but rather inositol hexanicotinate or niacinamide, a metabolic breakdown product of niacin but not the active ingredient that can lower lipids. Those products are flat-out fraud. Unfortunately, the FDA can't do much about them.

If you want a niacin product that is safe and clinically proven to be effective, with virtually no flush, get Endur-acin from Endurance Products. Doctors who have used it with their patients swear by it, and it works for me too.

COENZYME Q-10

Health food and drug store shelves are loaded with products that contain coenzyme Q10, either alone or in combination with other ingredients. It is typically listed as co-Q10. There's been so much hype over the years that this supplement's properties have reached nearly mythical status. True believers abound. They say it's "good for the heart." Too bad it doesn't work.

Co-Q10 is the common term for the chemical substance technically named ubiquinone. It got that name because it is ubiquitous, found in literally every organ of the body, especially those engaged in heavy activity such as the heart and lungs. Here are the truths: those tissues need co-Q10 to function properly, and co-Q10 levels tend to diminish with age. But it's also true that, regardless of age, we produce plenty of the stuff without the need for supplements.

First, co-Q10 has absolutely no effect on blood fats, including cholesterol. Second, although there was a glimmer of hope that the vitamin-like substance might improve heart muscle function in those with previous damage to the heart, carefully controlled research has now pulled the plug. Co-Q10 had absolutely no effect on those with heart failure, those most likely to have benefited from it.

Is it safe? Sure. It can do no harm, but does it do any good? Absolutely not. So save your money.

CHELATION THERAPY

Now we enter the arena of pure, unadulterated quackery. This is the worst kind of charlatanism, giving afflicted people false hope, taking away money many can ill afford to lose, and often delaying legitimate life-saving medical and surgical care.

Chelation therapy has a long history, beginning, as so many forms of quackery do, with legitimate applications for lead and mercury poisoning. When the chemcial EDTA is infused into the blood, it "chelates," or binds onto heavy metals. It has been used quite successfully for years to treat poisoning victims, often in industrial settings.

It was then reasoned that since calcium is a heavy metal, EDTA can chelate that as well. This was in the safe zone of truth. A later claim—that since calcium is a component of arterial plaque (especially in older, stabilized blockages), chelation therapy can bind onto that calcium, remove it from the plaque, and lead to disease regression—moved this theory into the fuzzy zone. There was even a book called *Bypassing Bypass,* which claimed that chelation eliminates the need for such surgery.

Sound good? Sure it does. It takes quite a bit of knowledge and understanding to detect the flaws in the argument. EDTA can indeed chelate calcium and remove it from the body. But it can only do so in the bloodstream, not in the established, hardened plaque that is actually within the layers of the artery. Calcium-laden plaque does not simply form on the inner wall of the artery like mineral buildup in a water pipe. It is impossible for the EDTA to get to the calcium in the plaque, much less chip it away like so much cruddy buildup in the plumbing.

Not one single, solitary research effort has shown any disease improvement. Not even when the EDTA infusion protocol has been approved by the "professional" organization of chelation therapists. The most definitive proof that chelation has no benefit over placebo came in the form of a study in which 84 patients with proven heart disease were given either chelation or "dummy" therapy. All received 30 "treatments" over 15 weeks, each lasting three hours. At the end of the study, there was no difference between "real" chelation and placebo. The study was published in the January 23, 2002 issue of the *Journal of the American Medical Association*.

Here's one time you can't trust people despite legitimate credentials. Chelation therapists are licensed physicians, and their clinics are staffed by registered nurses. These rogues are good salespersons, trotting out former patients, who provide excellent testimonials and who provide the aura of tender loving care we all crave.

Actually, doctors can and should learn from the chelation therapists and their staff members. Patients are greeted in the clinic by smiling faces and asked how they are feeling, and everyone seems to really care and to listen to complaints. A lot of touching and laying on of hands goes on in those offices. Patients are filled with trust and follow recommendations provided far more compliantly than those given by ordinary doctors. They are told and cajoled into quitting smoking, cutting back on saturated fats, and doing a lot of walking and other physical activity. They are often given (sold) "special" supplements that reinforce their confidence in the chelation sessions with every tablet and capsule swallowed. After several very costly visits to the clinic, they start feeling better. And they credit it all to chelation therapy and the "wonderful doctors and nurses" who "saved my life and kept me away from those scalpel-happy doctors."

In truth, it is the lifestyle modification patients achieve rather than the chelation therapy that makes them feel better. Sometimes making such changes, and thereby lowering cholesterol and blood pressure, will be sufficient to prevent progression of CHD. Of course, patients pay an enormous price for the "service."

But other times, going through the lengthy process of chelation therapy puts off needed testing and possibly surgery. Heart disease kills, and this is no time to put your health and your life in the hands of quacks.

ECCP: MORE FAKE THERAPY

The radio advertising and direct-mail promotions make ECCP sound like it's the latest medical breakthrough, fully clinically proven to relieve the symptoms of angina and reverse the progression of CHD. Clinics are popping up all over the country, and like the chelation clinics, they are staffed by people with medical credentials.

ECCP stands for extracorporeal counterpulsation. In a series of sessions, a contraption is wrapped around the legs that supposedly forces blood backward through the arteries in a rhythmic series of contractions beginning at the ankles and working its way up the leg. Advocates claim that the therapy results in the formation of so-called collateral circulation, with tiny new blood vessels springing up and branching from the coronary arteries.

As with other kinds of charlatanism, ECCP begins with some scientific truth. The body is definitely capable of forming those collateral arteries. That happens over many years of gradual progression of coronary heart disease. In fact, the *only* way collaterals form is as a response to gradual blockage of the coronary arteries.

Promoters of ECCP say that patients can cause the formation of collateral circulation through regular, strenuous exercise, forcing blood through the arteries at higher pressure than normal. ECCP, they say, mimics that exercise and speeds up the process. In fact, their entire case is built on the idea that exercise leads to collateral circulation.

But that premise is incorrect. It is a common medical myth that exercise can form collaterals. Many health professionals believe it to be true since it's often repeated, but while there are all sorts of other good reasons to exercise, it does *not* establish collateral circulation. Again, the only way collaterals can form is over a long period of gradual progression of disease in the arteries. It is the body's way of doing its own natural bypass to provide the heart muscle with additional blood flow.

I have spoken with experts from major medical centers—the Cleveland Clinic, UCLA, and Emory University—and all agree that ECCP is worthless, despite promoters' claims and clients' testimonials.

And contrary to the promotors' claims, it's not even new, much less revolutionary. ECCP has been around for a couple of decades. Originally it was used for patients with congestive heart failure. Again, there is no clinical evidence that ECCP works to improve the heart's circulation.

WHY DO WORTHLESS MEASURES THRIVE?

If this supplement or that therapy doesn't work, how does it survive on the market? And why do people swear that it works wonders?

We've already seen one reason in the chelation and ECCP clinics: Beneficial results are not the result of the therapy but rather of the lifestyle changes therapists encourage. The same is often true for various supplements.

Here's one great example. A company markets a weight loss potion that is to be drunk at bedtime. It is said to result in weight loss "while you sleep." But read the directions and you will see that you must take it on an "empty stomach" and not eat anything after 8 P.M. See the trick? The potion is worthless—the weight loss comes from cutting calories.

Then there are the companies that employ distributors to sell products and enroll others. Those distributors attend regular "pep rally" sales meetings that convince them of the tremendous value of the products they are buying, using, and selling. Of course, the profit motive doesn't hurt either.

Finally, and most important, there is the placebo effect. Does something work because it really, truly has an effect on the body or because one believes it is having that effect? The power of mind over body is tremendous, and we are learning more about it all the time.

Every scientifically valid research study uses a control group, which gets a placebo in the exact same setting as the treatment group getting the active ingredient being tested. That way one can measure the differences in response in both groups.

But things aren't always what they seem. In any study, there are a number of participants who drop out owing to adverse reactions or side effects. But quite often investigators find that as many suffer ill effects from the placebo as from the active agent. If a person hears that a pill may cause gastric upset, digestive problems may occur whether the pill is real or fake. Conversely, many of those getting the placebo improve. In the case of drugs meant to alter mental states in some way, or to help one sleep, the placebo can equal, or almost equal, the effectiveness of the drug.

My dad was a pharmacist in Chicago. He occasionally got prescriptions for sugar pills for doctors whose patients insisted on medication. One time I remember his conversation with a physician who instructed him to charge a particular patient more money than Dad thought was justified. The doctor explained that the patient was wealthy and could easily afford the fee and wouldn't think the "medicine" was any good unless it was expensive.

Today we have companies selling supplements at exorbitant prices, claiming that their products have superior properties. Because the price is high, people believe that effectiveness must also be greater than their generic counterparts.

A physician's attitude also influences the success of a medication he or she prescribes. If it is given with confidence and authority, such as "I'm sure this will fix you up quickly, I've been using it for years," the medication will be more effective than if the doctor waffles with something like "We can try this, but I'm not sure it will work in your case."

SEPARATING THE WHEAT FROM THE CHAFF

How do you make a decision regarding a service or product? How can you tell if something is legitimate or fake? We live in a country that provides tremendous latitude to companies and individuals through our freedom of speech, so you must do your homework.

Find out what proof exists that something works or is good for you. Has the research been conducted in a reputable institution? Were the results published in a credible journal after review by authorities in the field who have no personal involvement or vested interest? Have those results been replicated in subsequent studies done at other institutions by other scientists?

Always consider the source. Would you expect a used-car salesman to point out all the problems in an automobile he's trying to sell? Why would you expect anything more from a person or company trying to sell you a pill? Don't take anyone's word for anything. Demand proof.

Now you might just be asking yourself, "Why should I believe you, Bob?"

Good question. Will I profit if you decide to buy oat bran or beans at the supermarket? No. Will I get a check in the mail if you start taking the niacin I recommend? No. Do I provide scientific documentation for the things I say? Yes. Check out the references for yourself, provided at the end of the book.

Most important, will I feel like a million dollars if you follow my recommendations, start feeling better, have improved cholesterol tests, and write me a letter as thousands of men and women have already done over the years? You bet! I truly feel that this is my mission in life—to help you fight heart disease. Want to write that letter? Send it to me at PO Box 2039, Venice, CA 90294. I would love to hear from you.

10
Take Your Heart Out for a Walk

Way back in the mid-1980s when I submitted my manuscript for *The 8-Week Cholesterol Cure*, the editor asked why I wanted to include a chapter on exercise in a book targeting cholesterol. I thought it was quite obvious, and I still do. Physical activity remains an essential component of a heart-healthy lifestyle, and it also affects cholesterol levels.

Shortly before the book's publication in 1987, the Gallup Organization found in a poll that 54 percent of the entire population did some form of exercise. Sadly, as we've learned more about the enormous benefits of physical activity, that number has declined. Today, with sedentary behavior recognized as a major heart disease risk factor, only 22 percent of us get the recommended amount of exercise; 60 percent of the poulation is completely sedentary—true couch potatoes. Each year, 250,000 men and women die because of sedentary behavior.

How far would you walk, run, bicycle, or swim to save another person's life? Or would you just sit on the sofa and let that person die? Years ago, a cigarette advertisement spoke of walking a mile for a Camel. Is your heart—your life—not worth more than a cigarette?

My files bulge with research articles documenting the many health benefits of regular physical activity. Here are the reasons you and I must get out of that chair and show our hearts we really care.

First of all, you'll feel better. No kidding. Promise to give it a try for just 90 days. Sort of like trying one of those products on TV infomercials. Except that this one costs nothing and after that 90-day trial you won't want to return it to go back to your old ways. You'll have more energy, more get-up-and-go. You'll sleep better, and you'll enjoy life at an amazingly improved level.

Second, just about every heart disease risk factor will be significantly improved. Literally hundreds of research studies detail how exercise lowers LDL, total cholesterol, and triglycerides, normalizes blood pressure, maintains healthy weight, and more. Here are just a few details.

- The higher the level of fitness, the fewer beats your heart needs per minute to pump blood to the body and to the heart muscle itself. The average person's heart beats 72 times per minute. Physical conditioning will easily lower that number into the 60s and, with a little more effort, into the 50s.
- A regular program of physical activity along with some dietary changes can bring mild to moderate elevations in blood pressure down as well as prescription drugs. Reductions of blood pressure persist many hours after even a single exercise session.
- Exercise promotes the development of lean muscle tissue and decreases percentages of body fat. Those changes, in turn, lead to increases in the levels of the protective HDL cholesterol. Triglycerides also go down.
- Activity is an essential component of any weight loss program and vital for keeping off those pounds. Researchers at the Harvard School of Public Health found that regular exercise dramatically lowered levels of the "fat hormone" leptin. Made by the body's fat cells, leptin is believed to be a major culprit in causing obesity.
- A study published in the *New England Journal of Medicine* in February 2000 showed how exercise makes the arteries themselves healthier. Those engaged in routine physical exercise were rewarded by toning up the endothelium, the inner lining of the arteries. The more pliant and elastic the endothelium, the more easily the arteries can open up to allow for greater blood flow.
- Heart attacks are frequently the result of a blood clot that blocks the flow of blood to the heart's muscle. Those who regularly exercise have lower levels of fibrinogen, a substance that precipitates clots, and higher levels of fibrinolysis, the process of dissolving clots before they do any damage.
- Exercise is one of the greatest stress-busters. It takes a leap of faith to go out for a brisk, 15-minute walk rather than, say, grabbing a candy bar or a martini and plopping down on the couch, but of all the possible choices, exercise will make you less tense and more capable of dealing with the pressures of everyday life.
- You'll be more productive at work. Most people feel sleepy by midafternoon. Those who exercise regularly find that midday

letdowns are a thing of the past. In a survey of highly successful men and women in a number of professions, Dr. Kenneth Pelletier of Stanford University found that virtually all had a regular schedule of physical activity and that they credited their productivity to their exercise habits. Who knows? Maybe you'll even wind up making more money!

- You'll prevent heart attacks. Do at least two hours of vigorous activity weekly and you can reduce your risk of having a heart attack by as much as 70 percent.

- The benefits of physical activity accrue even when other risk factors such as obesity, smoking, elevated cholesterol levels, and others are present. Of course, all those risk factors tend to be ameliorated as exercise becomes routine.

- You'll enjoy your leisure time more. Today's PGA golfers, for example, depend on physical training to keep their scores down. No matter what your game or sport, ability and enjoyment perk up with exercise.

- Oh, by the way, you'll live longer. No, it won't just feel that way. Major studies have proven this "incidental" side effect of regular physical activity. And this is one time when if a little is good, more is better. The more you exercise, and the more strenuous that exercise is, the longer you will live.

Moreover, it's not only a matter of quantity of life but also of quality. Exercise can truly make those senior years, and all the years in between now and then, golden.

Look around you. Notice the men and women who seem much younger than their years. They have more energy, get more things done, and seem a lot happier. They also seem to get sick less often and have fewer aches and pains that limit their activities. Nine times out of ten, you'll find that those men and women make physical activity a way of life, getting in some exercise of one kind or another on a regular basis, probably several days a week.

IT'S NEVER TOO LATE

There's a law of physics called the "moment of inertia." That refers to the energy needed to start, for example, a boulder rolling down a mountain. At first it takes a lot of effort, but once that boulder gets going, it's almost impossible to stop.

If you're truly sedentary, preferring to remain motionless on the couch or in the easy chair, you're like that boulder. At first it might seem impossible to get active. But as with all worthwhile efforts, once you get going, activity becomes easier and easier. And like that boulder, you'll start a landslide of benefits and you won't want to quit.

Believe me, I've been there. I've never been the athletic type, preferring books to sports as a child. In fact, I was always the last one picked for any school games in physical education class, and I failed the President's Fitness Test back in the 1950s. In college I hung around with the academic types rather than the jocks, and after graduation I didn't even have classes to walk to. I became totally sedentary.

After my heart attack and first bypass operation, the doctors simply told me to "take it easy." Those were the days before cardiac rehabilitation and regular exercise for heart patients. I am sure that my inactivity contributed to the progression of my atherosclerosis and subsequent need for a second surgery.

But that's when my life really changed. Being "forced" into cardiac rehab in 1984 at the age of 41, I saw patients in their sixties and seventies walking energetically on the treadmill or cycling strenuously on their stationary bikes. I realized I couldn't keep up with them. Besides, they were happy, chatting and smiling, and that made me think, "Maybe there is something to all of this."

By the end of the 12-week rehab period, I was going strong. Impressed by the progress I'd made and how well I felt—better than I'd felt in years—I signed up for another 12 weeks. That led to a membership in a local health club, and I've been working out ever since. One day the treadmill, walking at an incline. Another day it might be the rowing machine or Stairmaster.

Today, in my late fifties, I have more energy and vitality than I did in my sedentary thirties. I can work longer hours, without that midday letdown. I sleep like a log. And I perform better at sports such as golf and skiing. I revel in that physical and psychological boost I get from a good workout. Doctors explain it in terms of the neurotransmitter beta-endorphin, but I think of it as a natural high. And if an injury or illness keeps me inactive for more than a few days, I actually miss my exercise. I quickly start feeling out-of-sorts, lethargic, and irritable.

Please believe me that I say all of this not to boast but to encourage you. It is truly never too late to start. You'll start reaping the benefits of feeling better almost immediately. Thousands and thousands of like-minded people can't all be wrong. And your heart will thank you for it. Research has demonstrated that physical activity at any age forestalls the onset and progression of coronary artery disease. The most active men and women in the famous Framingham Heart Study had a 40 percent lower overall mortality rate during 16 years of observation than did those in the least active third of the study population.

But wait. You say you were pretty athletic as a kid and through college. Or you were really active in your twenties and thirties and only started getting sedentary in your forties. Shouldn't that give you some protection? Sorry, but that's not the case.

In the Framingham Study, only *recent* exercise made a significant difference. Exercise done earlier in life showed no long-term protective effect. In a study of Harvard alumni, those who were now sedentary after having been college athletes had just as high a risk of heart disease as those who had always been sedentary. Conversely, alumni who were previously inactive and got back to physical activity slashed their risk. When it comes to your heart, it's a question of "What have you done for me lately?"

Moreover, you are never (that's right—*never*) too old to begin an active lifestyle. At first that might merely mean walking up a flight of stairs rather than using the elevator or parking the car a block away from your destination and walking the rest of the way. That might lead to daily walks up and down the block. Eventually, you'll surprise yourself pleasantly and increase that activity to walking a mile or two daily. Take it one step at a time.

In a study called the Honolulu Heart Program, doctors worked with 2678 physically active men aged 71 to 93 years. During a four-year period, 109 men developed coronary heart disease. Men who walked less than a quarter of a mile a day had twice the risk of those who walked more than a mile and a half a day. Although risk declined for those walking somewhere between that quarter mile and the mile and a half, the really dramatic decrease in risk occurred with men who walked the most.

I take great personal pride in the fact that I can often run (or at least walk) circles around men half my age. It's not just a "guy thing." Women I've spoken with feel the same way. And there's proof that our arteries can perform as well as those of the "youngsters."

Researchers studied sedentary individuals and athletes, young and old. Athletes included runners, cyclists, and swimmers. Both groups of young people, sedentary and athletic, averaged 27 years of age. The average ages for the older groups were 63 for the sedentary folks and 66 for the athletic types. Doctors found that the older athletes' blood vessels functioned as well as those of both the active and sedentary younger men.

So why care about our blood vessels? In healthy arteries the lining (endothelium) produces a substance called nitric oxide (NO) that helps the vessels dilate when the heart needs more blood. NO also protects the vessel walls from developing atherosclerosis, the buildup of crud that blocks the flow of blood, and thrombosis, the formation of blood clots that can block small or narrowed vessels and cause heart attacks. As we age, the endothelium produces less NO, making older individuals more prone to atherosclerosis and thrombosis. But regular physical activity can prevent and even reverse the aging of the endothelium.

Nitric oxide produced by the endothelium affects *all* our arteries, not just those in the heart. When NO production drops, the arteries are less able to pump blood and oxygen to the various parts of our bodies. That includes the penis. In fact, the drug Viagra works by increasing NO production, allowing more blood flow to the penis. So, guys, regular exercise can and will improve that part of your lives as well! And ladies, you will find that your enjoyment increases with physical activity as well.

HOW OFTEN AND HOW MUCH?

"It's not that I don't want to exercise, but I just don't have time." That's the objection I hear most. And when some people describe their days, it's difficult to argue that they can fit in another hour or so to go to the gym. No problem.

Certainly it's nice to be able to head off for a long hike in the woods, a two-hour bicycle ride, or a leisurely workout at the health club followed by relaxing in the sauna. But for the man or woman who gets up at 5:30 A.M. to commute to work and doesn't get back home until 7 P.M., that's just not likely to happen. Fortunately, physical activity doesn't have to come in one big chunk to provide heart benefits.

Years ago, health authorities recited the "30 minutes" mantra: exercise had to last a minimum of 30 minutes to be of any benefit. In fact, I heard one doctor say that if one was on a treadmill or stationary bicycle at home for, say, 7 minutes, and then stopped to answer the phone, the clock went back to zero and one would have to start all over to get in a full 30 minutes of uninterrupted exercise. Sadly, I heard that doctor give that advice just last year. He simply wasn't up to speed on the latest exercise research.

Studies were first done at Stanford University that showed that breaking up the total day's physical activity into smaller bites could be just as good as continuous exercise. That was about ten years ago. Then in 1997, researchers examined the data of more than 22,000 men enrolled in a long-term study of physicians' health behaviors. They found that if you don't have time for a 30-minute workout each day, it's just as good to divide the time into much shorter periods of activity. As frequency of exercise increased from one to five days weekly, risk of heart attack and death from heart disease declined. The men who exercised five or more times a week had 46 percent fewer heart attacks than those who exercised less often than once a week.

In 2000, results from a comparable study of female nurses revealed equal benefits for women. That same year, the American Heart Association published data showing that short sessions lasting about 15 minutes provide cumulative benefits. It all adds up to protect your heart.

You can fit physical activity into even the most hectic and stressful day. In fact, periodic exercise is one of the best ways to cope with modern stress and pressures on the job. Instead of taking that 15-minute break in the morning to drink coffee and eat doughnuts, neither of which does your heart any good, go out for a brisk walk, swinging your arms back and forth. You'll come back to the office feeling refreshed, relaxed, and ready for the job ahead. Then, at the end of the day, park the car in the garage and take another 15-minute walk. A lot of people now bring athletic shoes to change into for those "vitality breaks."

But what about intensity? Must one engage in extremely strenuous exercise with sweat spraying and tongue hanging out? Absolutely not. Although some people truly enjoy long, exhausting jogging or other activities, it's definitely not necessary.

In the first place, it's simply not practical to expect a person in his fifites, sixties, or seventies to go from decades of almost total inactivity to superathlete status. And regardless of age, most people do not want to—or physcially cannot—attain that level of fitness. Moreover, as physical activity becomes more extreme, the chances of injury increase.

So what is enough exercise? There are two ways of answering that question. On a simple level, if your exercise is walking, do so as though you are in a hurry to get to your destination at a speed that gets your heart beating faster and makes you breathe harder. The same applies to other activities. On a more scientific level, you want to boost your metabolism to a point where your entire body, as well as your heart, is expending more energy. Scientists measure this work in metabolic equivalents of task (METs). The more active the task, the higher the number of METs. Sitting in a chair or lying down on a couch takes just a little energy to keep the body functioning. That energy is calculated as 1 MET. Get up from that chair and walk to the kitchen for a snack, and you've increased your body's activity level to 2 METs. Virtually every human activity can be measured in terms of METs. Take a look at Table 8 to see how many METs are achieved by a wide variety of activities, from playing the piano to gardening to playing a competitive game of racquetball or jogging at least 6 miles per hour.

The chart will probably make you smile because you already do a lot of the activities listed. We are all active to one degree or another. The trick is to get our bodies burning more energy, putting out more METs more often. It's all about activity rather than strictly defined exercise.

As Table 8 reveals, walking at 3 miles per hour takes the same amount of effort, 3 to 4 METs, as heavier housework such as scrubbing dishes. Boost that walking stride to 4 miles per hour, 4 to 5 METs, and you're up to the equivalent of mowing the lawn with a power mower. Trade that in for a push-model mower and you climb to 6 to 7 METs, the same as walking at a speed of 5 miles per hour, which most folks can't do.

So whether you're actively working, playing, or doing specific exercise, you're achieving the same effect of upping the body's energy expenditure. Depending on your own personal capabilities and limitations, aim for doing a minimum of 30 minutes of daily activities in the range of 3 to 7 METs. Remember that is a *minimum*. If you can do more, terrific. Several research studies have shown that the more vigorous the activity, done for greater lengths of time, the greater the heart protection.

Here's another way at looking at how even bits and pieces of activity add up. Walking up and down a flight of 10 stairs burns 14 calories; do that every day and in a week you've burned 98 calories. Keeping all other exercise and calorie consumption equal, in 35 days you will have lost 1 pound of body weight just by walking that daily flight of stairs.

With walking, 1 mile burns at least 100 calories, depending on your weight. It's the same whether you walk that mile in 15 minutes or 20 minutes; you'll still have done the same amount of "work," achieving the same goal. Doing that mile daily incinerates many calories for the week. Make it 2 miles and you've gone through quite a few calories weekly, rather than staying sedentary. That additional caloric expenditure can result in a significant weight loss over time, all other things being equal. It's no wonder people who remain relatively active are seldom overweight. The more one exercises, the easier it is to maintain a healthy weight.

Table 8. **ENERGY REQUIREMENTS OF COMMON ACTIVITIES IN METS***

1 MET:	Sleeping, lying in bed, sitting quietly in a chair
2 METs:	Standing, talking, walking (1 mph), reading, writing, playing cards, light housekeeping (dusting), typing or word processing, shaving, dressing, or brushing hair
2–3 METs:	walking (2 mph), playing piano, playing golf (electric cart), bathing or showering, washing hair, moderate housekeeping (light laundry), meal preparation, bicycling (5 mph), bowling
3–4 METs:	walking (3 mph), bicycling (6–7 mph), driving a car in light traffic, climbing stairs slowly, heavier housework (scrubbing dishes), ballroom dancing (fox-trot), factory labor
4–5 METs:	walking (4 mph), bicycling (8 mph), gardening or raking, light carpentry, mowing lawn (power), playing badminton or light tennis, heavy housekeeping (mopping, vacuuming), house painting, driving a car in heavy traffic, washing windows
5–6 METs:	walking (4.5 mph), bicycling (10 mph), roller-skating, light shoveling, digging, golfing (carrying or pulling clubs), very heavy housework (scrubbing floors), carrying wood or groceries, social dancing (tango)
6–7 METs:	walking (5 mph), bicycling (11 mph), playing tennis (singles), waterskiing, swimming leisurely, mowing lawn (push mower), square dancing, splitting wood, snow shoveling, moving furniture
7–8 METs:	jogging (5 mph), bicycling (12 mph), downhill skiing, canoeing, swimming laps (slow), playing football, horseback riding at gallop, climbing hills (moderate), climbing stairs (continuous), playing tennis (competitive singles)
8–9 METs:	jogging (5.5 mph), bicycling (13 mph), swimming laps (fast), cross-country skiing, playing basketball, carrying groceries upstairs
10+ METs:	handball, racquetball, squash, climbing hills with a load, jogging (6 mph and faster)

*One MET equals the amount of energy needed when the body is at rest.
Two METs equal twice the amount of energy used when at rest.

Is there a point of diminishing returns when it comes to protecting your heart with exercise? Is more always better? Nope. Dr. Kenneth Cooper, the man who put the word "aerobics" into the English language many years ago, determined that the optimal level of exercise would be 15 miles weekly. Subsequent studies have come to the same conclusion.

You can do those 15 miles, or the equivalent, any way you prefer. You can walk briskly, you can jog, you can run. You can do a little over 2 miles a day. Or 3 miles a day for five days each week. Or 5 miles a day three days a week. It makes no difference.

Are there any advantages of doing more than 15 miles weekly? You might get some competitive satisfaction. You might want to get into top physical condition for the upcoming sports season. But as far as your heart's concerned, 15 miles is enough.

Conversely, the more *vigorously* you exercise, the better. Heart rate goes down along with blood pressure and triglycerides, and levels of protective HDL go up. Start walking to the best of your ability. Work your way up to managing 15 miles weekly. Then, if you want to do your heart more good, walk those miles more quickly. Or do so either on a treadmill at elevation or by walking up hills. Or put on a backpack and gradually add some weight to it, increasing the intensity of the walking experience.

Here's a terrific approach developed at Laval University in Quebec, Canada. It applies whether you're walking, bicycling, climbing stairs, or whatever. Each time you exercise, push it to the max for 30 to 90 seconds, then slow down for a while and repeat the process. The first time out, you might be able to do that only three or four times during a 30-minute period. The same applies even if you're doing a "quicky" 10 or 15 minutes. You'll be amazed at how you'll progress rapidly and at how much more satisfying the workout becomes. And you'll get an additional bonus for your efforts. Boosting the intensity by doing those 30-to-90-second bursts increases the time your body's metabolism remains elevated after the exercise period is over and done. In other words, you'll be burning more calories even when sitting at your desk or lounging in front of the TV for the rest of the evening. Not bad, huh?

WHAT'S THE BEST ACTIVITY?

Ultimately, the best physical activity is the one you do on a regular basis. For some people, like former President Reagan, it meant doing some strenuous work on the ranch. Don't have a ranch to clear of brush? Gardening and lawn mowing in your own backyard can be just as effective, and millions of people love to garden. Even heavy housework can provide the physical activity needed for the day.

Some people like going to the gym. It's a way of scheduling your activity, being in a place far from the phone and fax, and enjoying the companionship of others. I'm in that camp myself. For me it's a way of getting off to a good start and I feel refreshed and energized, ready for a day's work.

Five days a week, Monday through Friday, I do about 45 minutes of cardiovascular exercise on a variety of machines, including the treadmill, stairs, and rowing machine. My wife finds that routine totally dull and boring and prefers to take various aerobics classes in the evening after work. She likes being part of a group and has favorite instructors who take her through her paces.

Morning, afternoon, or evening? It really doesn't matter and is more of a personal preference. Do what you prefer and you will be more likely to stick with it.

But obviously the gym is not the choice for everyone. The idea of driving somewhere, checking in, getting a locker, getting on a machine, and walking, climbing, or rowing for an hour seems ridiculous to some people. So why not just go out for a walk or run?

If you're a jogger or runner and enjoy the experience and the "high" you get, terrific. But I don't recommend running unless you are already into it. Running is tough on the body, and inevitably, almost all runners get injured. What you want is something you can do and enjoy for the rest of your life. That's walking.

If walking could be "packaged" for a television infomercial, the claims would be extravagant and justified. Easy to begin, even for those who have not done exercise for decades. Very inexpensive, all you need is a good pair of walking shoes. Convenient, you can walk anywhere at any time. It's very pleasant and a walk can take you through the woods on a beautiful autumn day or down the streets of a new town or city you are visiting. It's very safe and about the only way to get injured is to be hit by a truck while crossing the street. Effective, walking provides all the exercise your heart will ever need, now and for the rest of your life. That last phrase rings an important bell. Unlike other activities, this is something everyone can do into his or her golden years. And there are hundreds of studies to back all this up. Here are just a few examples:

- Women in the Nurses' Health Study who walked the equivalent of three or more hours per week at a brisk pace slashed their risk of coronary events by 30 to 40 percent. That was about the same risk reduction achieved by those who engaged in regular vigorous exercise such as jogging or running or bouts in the gym. And women who became active in middle adulthood or later still had a lower risk than those who remained sedentary.

■ In the Honolulu Heart Study, men aged 61 to 81 were tracked for 12 years. Those who walked more than 2 miles daily had significantly lower mortality than those who walked less than 1 mile a day.

■ People participating in the Harvard University Alumni Study also demonstrated the wonderful benefits of walking. Those walking a 1-hour brisk walk, five days a week, had a 46 percent lower risk of stroke than those who did little or no exercise.

A brisk walk is defined for research purposes as walking at a pace anywhere from 3.0 to 3.9 miles per hour. Walking at a rate of 4.0 miles per hour or more is considered very brisk or strenuous. How fast do you walk? Measure the distance from, say, your house or office to a given point on your car's odometer. Then walk the distance and see how long it takes you to cover a mile. That's your pace.

Now a word to younger readers who might be thinking that all this is really aimed at the older folks. Think walking is not something for a truly fit person? Think again. Just about anyone in his or her twenties, thirties, or forties can run a mile in 10 or 12 minutes. How long you'll huff and puff afterward is another story. But try this test of fitness suggested by Swedish researchers. See if you can walk 2 miles in under 30 minutes. That's harder than you might imagine. And if you can cover those 2 miles in under 28 minutes, you're in excellent shape. Now try pushing it to do 3 miles at that 14-minute-mile pace.

Don't want to walk fast? Feel your legs are too short to go for speed? Take your walk to the hills or put the treadmill at an incline. That jacks up the MET level quickly. Another approach to getting your heart rate up is to follow the example of the Israeli army trainers. Start with a small backpack, the kind that kids take to school, and walk with it empty. Once you are comfortable with that, add a 5-pound bag of sugar to the backpack. Increase the weight as your fitness level rises. Using these tips, walking will never lack challenge, even for the most fit person.

Want to make walking a lot of fun? Do it on the golf course.

Finnish researchers proved that walking 18 holes of golf, either pulling or carrying the bag of clubs, two to three times a week offers the benefits of a structured exercise program. Weight, waist circumference, HDL cholesterol, and HDL-to-total cholesterol ratio were all improved.

IMPROVE MUSCLE TONE, HELP YOUR HEART

For years, the American Heart Association cautioned those diagnosed with heart disease against pumping iron, also known as weight training or resistance exercise. Then in February 2000, the AHA published a scientific advisory for cardiologists and other physicians in their official journal *Circulation*, reversing their position and actively advocating weight training. This was based on a tremendous body of evidence showing the benefits for everyone.

Please don't roll your eyes or turn the page. We're not talking about heavy-duty workouts in a sweaty gym surrounded by huge guys with tattoos. It's a matter of toning one's muscles to prevent typical degeneration associated with aging and improving a number of heart-health parameters. Blood pressure, cholesterol levels, weight, and blood sugar levels all improve with a bit of weight training.

The AHA calls for exercises that can be easily done at home, even in front of the TV. They recommend a single set of eight to ten different exercises that train the major muscle groups, done two to three times weekly. (Other research has shown that one day of weight training provides 70 percent of the benefits attained in two or three days. It would be best to do the exercises two to three days weekly, but if you just can't, one day a week will still help.)

Start with very light weights, perhaps dumbbells of only 2 or 3 pounds—5 pounds if you can handle it. You can pick up a set of dumbbells of varying weights in any sporting goods store very inexpensively. They typically come with instructions showing how you do the AHA-recommended exercises, which include chest press, shoulder press, triceps extension, biceps curl, pull-downs, lower-back extensions, abdominal crunches, quadriceps extensions, leg curls, and calf raises. Sound intimidating? It really isn't, and these exercises merely involve moving your body's muscles in various ways while holding the weights to provide resistance (hence the term "resistance training"). You'll be amazed at how quickly you notice improvement.

The National Institute on Aging offers two free publications. One is *Exercise: Feeling Fit for Life*. The other is a 100-page booklet,

Exercise: A Guide from the National Institute on Aging. To order, call 800-222-2225.

Think you're too old to start such foolishness? A study done at Tufts University proves you wrong. Researchers there worked with people in their nineties who had been almost completely sedentary. Those elderly men and women could scarcely get out of a chair without assistance. After a few weeks, they were rejuvenated, able to do things they hadn't been capable of in years. It was like finding a fountain of youth.

STRETCH A BIT WHEN FINISHED

Ask any chiropractor what leads to most injuries and disabilities and almost certainly he or she will say it's a lack of flexibility. As we age, our bodies become stiffer and less flexible, and typical inactivity speeds the process. We can counteract such degeneration with simple, easy-to-do, and even enjoyable gentle stretches daily. Take a cat as your role model as it awakens from a nap by stretching its body this way and that.

You can get illustrated instructions for stretching exercises from a chiropractor's office, at the YMCA, at the local hospital, in pharmacies, or even on videotape at the library or rental store.

After doing 10 or 15 minutes of stretching, you'll feel like you just had a nice massage. Be sure to stretch after any extended period of exercise, whether out for a long walk, at the gym, or golf or gardening.

BEFORE YOU START

Speak with your doctor if you haven't been active until now. Ask if he or she thinks you might have some limitations of any kind. This is especially true for those with exisiting heart disease resulting in symptoms of, say, chest pains (angina).

Wear appropriate clothing and comfortable, properly fitted shoes. By all means, don't overdo it at the beginning. Take baby steps. As the old Chinese proverb goes, the journey of a 1000 miles begins with a single step.

Along the way of that journey, get to know your heart on a "personal" basis. Tell your heart (silently so others won't think you're nuts) that you two are going out for a walk. As you go along, think of how your heart is pumping life-sustaining blood to every single part of your body. Feel it beating more rapidly as you pick up the pace. Know it's getting stronger with each step. Notice how you are breathing more heavily, sucking oxygen into your lungs for your heart to deliver to your body. Actively smile during your activity, reveling in the marvel of your body's movements. All this is known as active meditation. Such thoughts will make your exercise more enjoyable and contribute to the feeling of well-being you will have when you finish. Your heart will thank you for it by working for many years to come.

11
Sensible Solutions to Blood Pressure Control

About 60 million American adults have high blood pressure, a silent killer with no symptoms in nine out of ten cases. The only way to know if you have this problem is to have your pressure checked at your doctor's office or elsewhere. Hypertension is a major risk factor for cardiovascular disease, greatly increasing your chances of having a heart attack or stroke.

The really good news is that, working together with your physician, you can control your blood pressure. Mild to moderate cases of hypertension typically respond to lifestyle modifications. More severe blood pressure elevations may call for medication. One way or the other, getting your numbers down dramatically slashes your risk.

We don't think about blood pressure, since we can't feel it and there are no symptoms if it goes up. Even when calm and relaxed, pressure may be elevated. Over a period of time hypertension leads to a thickening or hardening of the arteries, which are also weakened in the process.

The first step is to understand that "blood pressure" refers to the pressure required to pump blood from the heart through the arteries to all parts of the body. Through a complex system of checks and balances, your body regulates and adjusts blood pressure.

There are two important blood pressure measurements. The first is the *systolic* pressure, that of the blood pushing against the artery wall as the heart beats. The second is the *diastolic* pressure, a measurement between beats when the heart rests. A reading of 120/80 is stated as "120 over 80." The systolic pressure is 120 and the diastolic is 80. That reading, by the way, is completely normal, and the patient would be termed "normotensive." A person whose pressure goes up is called "hypertensive."

Just a few years ago, doctors were particularly concerned about the lower, diastolic, pressure and often ignored the upper, systolic, number. Today we know that both pressures are important. In some cases, the diastolic pressure remains normal, but the systolic number goes up. That's called "isolated systolic hypertension" and should definitely be treated.

Here's a breakdown of blood pressure numbers for adults over 18. The measurements are in millimeters of mercury as seen in a column on the blood pressure machine (sphygmomanometer) when the doctor applies pressure and then releases it with a cuff around the arm.

Diastolic Blood Pressure	
Normal pressure	<85
High normal pressure	85– 89
Mild hypertension	90– 104
Moderate hypertension	105– 114
Severe hypertension	>160

Systolic Blood Pressure	
Normal pressure	<140
Borderline hypertension	140– 159
Severe hypertension	>160

Unless your pressure is way up, most doctors will hold off on medications for a while to see if some lifestyle modifications can bring it down. For a while, the ball is in your court, and it's up to you to improve your numbers sufficiently to avoid having to take drugs, which may have a number of adverse reactions.

There are some things we just can't do anything about as we age. Blood pressure tends to rise gradually. Certain ethnic groups, especially blacks, are at greater risk than others. But many factors can be modified. Research done within just the past few years dramatically demonstrates that mild to moderate hypertension responds very nicely to lifestyle changes. Just as with cholesterol, the lower we can get our numbers, the more we reduce our risk of cardiovascular disease.

Here are the things we know will work to reduce blood pressure:

- *Become more active.* If you've been sedentary, gradually ease into a lifestyle of daily physical activity. (See Chapter 10.)
- *Lose weight.* Overweight and obesity directly correlate with high blood pressure. I spell out the details on how to successfully attain a healthy weight in Chapter 12.
- *Limit alcohol consumption.* Those with severe hypertension may have to quit the booze entirely. Most can succeed simply

by cutting back to one drink a day, or perhaps to one drink a few times weekly.

- *Get rid of the cigarettes.* As a former smoker myself, I know it's tough to do, but millions of others have done it, and you can too. Your doctor will be happy to help you with nicotine patches or gum or antianxiety medications to get you through the toughest first weeks.

- *Control your stress.* We all have stress in our daily lives; the difference is that some men and women cope better than others. Take an active role. Find a stress-busting technique that works for you—perhaps biofeedback, or a hobby that gets your mind off day-to-day concerns. Physical activity really takes the edge off.

- *Get a pet.* Or spend more time with the one you already have in the family. Psychologists have demonstrated time and again that the simple act of stroking a dog or cat brings down blood pressure. Just having an animal in the room with you can be calming.

- *Make some dietary changes.* Eat more fruits and vegetables, especially those rich in potassium. Cut back on rich, fatty foods. The worst thing you can do is to have a big high-fat meal after a particularly stressful day.

- *Consider professional help.* No one thinks getting a personal trainer to start a program in the gym is unusual. We rely on brokers to help make investment decisions. Why not turn to an expert in stress or anger management? Your doctor can give you a referral.

Those are the lifestyle modifications that work best to control hypertension. And they're things that everyone can and should do to keep our numbers as low as possible, since even slight elevations over normal increase risk. Is there anything you've noticed that I've not included in the checklist? Yup, it's salt and sodium restriction.

For many people, reductions in sodium intake help control hypertension. That's because salt and other sodium compounds are involved in a chemical sequence initiated in the kidneys that ends with the production of a substance that raises blood pressure.

During the past couple of decades, we've heard the unequivocal advice that all Americans should significantly reduce their salt and sodium consumption. Few questioned the authorities, and salt was labeled "the enemy." It got to where no one dared to reach for the salt shaker in public.

I followed the "party line" on sodium in *The 8-Week Cholesterol Cure*. Then research data began to indicate sodium advice should be taken with the proverbial grain of salt. Not everyone's blood pressure fell even when sodium intake was severely restricted. My subsequent books and my quarterly publication *The Diet-Heart Newsletter* reflected the new thinking that not everyone should cut back radically on salt and sodium.

Wow, did I ever get blasted for that! It was as though I were living in the twelfth century and stood accused of heresy. During a presentation in Santa Monica in which I discussed the sodium issue, a person with the Pritikin Longevity Center loudly interrupted, saying that I was undermining good medical advice. Undaunted, I presented solid research data to back up my thoughts. And when the Pritikin representative continued to interrupt, the audience booed him down. That was in 1990.

Today the issue has become controversial in medical and scientific circles. Not everyone, not even major officials in the American Heart Association, believes that sodium reduction ought to be a universal goal for all Americans. Many are paying attention to the research data piling up in the medical literature and are concluding that, at the very least, old-line dogma ought to be changed.

Even before I get into some of the details as to why I don't think that sodium reduction is all it's cracked up to be, I need to offer a disclaimer. First, no one should consume unlimited quantities of salt and sodium. There's way too much in the typical American diet, largely owing to processed foods and typical fast foods. From a culinary point of view, not everything should taste as salty as brine from the olive jar. Second, some people are particularly sensitive to salt (more about that in just a bit) and must restrict it to achieve control of hypertension.

However, scientific facts have toppled public health theory. First, salt intake does not always lead to increased blood pressure unless taken to extremes. Second, only a small percentage of people are sodium-sensitive. Third, sodium restriction does not lower blood pressure for all people. Fourth, other minerals must be balanced, and at least one, potassium, is even more important in blood pressure control than sodium. Fifth, severe sodium restriction may actually be harmful for some individuals. Now let's look at these issues in some detail so we can come to logical rather than emotional conclusions.

The international Intersalt Study is the most comprehensive population study yet undertaken to get some answers to this controversy. Researchers looked at blood pressure and sodium intake in people in 32 countries. They found little link between the two. Only where sodium intakes were either extremely low or extremely high could one derive a statistical association. And statistical averages do not reflect individual differences. Some people get high blood pressure even on low-sodium diets, while others maintain normal pressures though their diets are high in sodium.

SODIUM SENSITIVITY

Some lucky people can eat all the wrong foods and still have a normal cholesterol count. And most people can enjoy sugar without developing diabetes, though those who have the metabolic disorder must carefully limit sugar intake. Similarly, not all men and women need to be overly restrictive when it comes to salt and sodium; in such cases, genes trump diet.

Yes, everyone's blood pressure will go up a few points if given an extreme amount of salt. But only those individuals with what is termed "salt sensitivity" will respond to moderate salt intake.

Doctors at the University of Utah actually identified the "salt gene" and reported their findings in the September 1998 issue of *Hypertension*. Technically called the angiotensinogen gene, this hereditary trait causes some individuals to make increased levels of the hormone angiotensinogen. Carriers of that gene respond dramatically to changes in dietary salt content. Tests for the salt gene are not yet commonly available.

Just because your current blood pressure is normal doesn't necessarily mean that you are not salt-sensitive, since pressure problems develop slowly as we age. That's why some authorities stick with the old recommendation that the entire population should cut back on salt. This approach will, they say, help those who would develop hypertension later in life, and does no harm or causes no major deprivation for those who would remain normotensive regardless of diet. There are quite a few kinks in that reasoning.

LOW-SALT DIETS CAN CAUSE HARM

Ironically, reducing sodium intake for those with existing hypertension can actually result in raising blood pressure rather than lowering it. Doctors have to be very careful in monitoring patients. As the ancient Hippocratic oath states, "First, do no harm."

Dr. Brent Egan, then at the Medical College of Wisconsin, found that a low-salt diet did not reduce blood pressure in 50 percent of patients with hypertension and had no effect on 80 percent of those with normal blood pressures. For some people, the diet switch caused pressures to rise.

Even more disturbing, Dr. Michael Alderman at the Albert Einstein College of Medicine in New York City linked low sodium consumption with an increase in heart attack risk! His study followed nearly 2000 men for almost four years. More than four times as many heart attacks occurred in men with the lowest amounts of sodium in their diets, as determined by the amount of sodium found in the urine.

Such findings don't mean that everyone should gobble pickles and olives and salt their food until it's white. But they do cast a big dark shadow on blanket recommendations for the entire U.S. population.

LOW-SALT DIETS OFTEN DO NOT WORK

Spurred by admonitions from professional organizations, including the American Heart Association and the American Medical Association, doctors tell their patients to cut back on salt and sodium in rather a knee-jerk fashion. If such restrictions did some good, they'd be worth the deprivation and lesser enjoyment of food. Some patients actually become obsessed and neurotic, viewing a salt shaker like a loaded gun pointed at their heads. But the research published in the AMA's and the AHA's own official journals don't justify blanket recommendations.

Here's the conclusion of one research team in 1996, published in the *Journal of the American Medical Association:* reduced dietary sodium resulted in "decreases in blood pressure that were larger in trials of older hypertensive individuals and small and nonsignificant in trials of normotensive individuals." That was their finding after reviewing 56 separate hypertension trials and pooling the results, in what is called a meta-analysis.

And in May 1998, *JAMA* published the conclusions of another group summarizing the effects of efforts to control hypertension with sodium restriction. "These results do not support a general recommendation to reduce sodium intake."

No less than the American Heart Association's past president, Dr. Suzanne Oparil, agrees. Unfortunately, she was unable to modify the AHA's rigid stance.

WHAT SHOULD YOU DO ABOUT SALT?

For a while I believed that if one has a normal blood pressure there is no need to do anything beyond moderating dietary salt and sodium intake. "If it ain't broke, don't fix it." But such individuals might indeed be salt-sensitive and could develop hypertension gradually as they age. At the other end of the spectrum those with existing hypertension owe it to themselves and those they love to make a solid effort to cut back on sodium. But in all cases, the question to be answered is, "Am I salt-sensitive, and will cutting back on sodium decrease my blood pressure?" Consider yourself a guinea pig in an absolutely crucial experimental trial.

So, no matter what your blood pressure currently is, test yourself. Get a reading in your doctor's office or at the pharmacy. You might even consider purchasing a home blood pressure monitor. These fully automated devices have been clinically tested and found to be just as accurate as a test with a stethoscope and sphygmomanometer in the doctor's office. A good one is the Omron HEM-705CP; Sunbeam also makes accurate monitors. Whichever you buy, have it tested for accuracy at your doctor's office. He or she will be pleased to see you taking an active role in your own care.

With the initial blood pressure reading as a baseline, cut back on salt and sodium. Read the labels on processed and commercially baked foods. Ease up on the salt shaker. Limit the amount of fast foods you eat.

If you decide on a home monitor, check your pressure daily and keep a written record. If not, see if a local pharmacy offers a blood pressure testing machine, or have the nurse at your doctor's office measure your pressure at one-week intervals. Mark down the results. Within one month, you'll know whether you respond to and benefit from sodium restriction. If you see an improvement, you'll cut your risk of stroke and heart attack by keeping it up. As time goes on, your tastebuds will adapt quickly, and soon you won't miss the salt.

On the other hand, if you don't see any blood pressure changes, or if they are insignificant, you've learned that you are not salt-sensitive. That doesn't mean you should go hog-wild with salt and sodium. Rather, practice moderation. Even if it doesn't affect your blood pressure, excessive sodium can lead to water retention.

You'll derive other benefits as well. Fast food not only has a lot of salt but is also loaded with saturated and trans fats. The same goes for many commercially prepared processed foods, including soups, TV dinners, and baked goods. Put Nutrition Facts labels at the top of your must-read list.

IF NOT SODIUM, THEN WHAT?

For most people, sodium is the wrong mineral to be concerned about. Instead of worrying about consuming too much sodium, pay more attention to potassium, magnesium, and calcium.

For years, Dr. David McCarron has researched the link between calcium and hypertension and has lobbied, with only partial success, to convince authorities and the public to turn to calcium-rich dairy and other foods rather than simply turning away from the salt shaker. The physician from the Oregon Health Sciences University points to connections between low calcium intake and increased arterial pressure. Pregnant women reduce both their systolic and diastolic blood pressure when they take calcium supplements. Men and women who improve their all-around diet, thereby ensuring adequate regular consumption of calcium, potassium, and magnesium, show more impressive improvements in blood pressure than those who take the negative approach of restricting sodium. And studies that have focused on calcium specifically have shown pressure reductions when calcium intake goes up, although the improvements are not dramatic.

Similarly, patients given magnesium supplements have shown a small but significant improvement. Researchers speculate that magnesium may play a role in relaxing the blood vessels. When arteries are constricted rather than relaxed and supple, the heart works harder to pump blood, thereby causing blood pressure to increase. Magnesium supplements worked best for those with more than slightly elevated blood pressure.

Potassium has taken the center stage as the mineral star in hypertension control. The body works to keep a balance of potassium and sodium. If your diet is high in potassium, you will excrete more sodium in your urine; conversely, a large intake of sodium can lead to increases in potassium loss.

Several different research studies have pointed to the value of increasing potassium intake. In one investigation of nearly 44,000 men, individuals in the top fifth of dietary potassium intake had a 38 percent lower risk of stroke than those in the bottom fifth. In that study, potassium came from fruit and vegetable consumption. Another study focusing on women's risk of hypertension found that potassium improved both systolic and diastolic pressures; again the mineral came from a diet rich in fruits and vegetables. But a third study got similar or even better results when potassium supplements were given to patients. In all cases, the higher blood pressure is to begin with, the greater improvements seen with potassium.

When doctors at Johns Hopkins University combined and reviewed the results of 33 different trials looking at the effects of potassium on blood pressure, the results were very positive. For those with hypertension, the mineral lowered systolic pressure by 4.4 points, and diastolic pressure by 2.5 points on average. Those with normal pressures to begin with saw more modest improvements of 3.1 systolic and 2.0 diastolic. Doctors have suggested a target intake of about 1600 mg of potassium daily. Table 9 shows that this is not a difficult goal to reach.

Table 9. **SOURCE OF POTASSIUM**

Food	Amount	Potassium (Mg)
Honeydew melon	¼ melon	940
Potato (baked)	1 medium	844
Dried figs	5 whole	666
Prunes	10 medium	626
Dates	10 whole	541
Tomato puree	½ cup	525
Dried apricots	10 halves	482
Banana	1 medium	451
Winter squash	½ cup	445
Raisins	⅓ cup	375
Lima beans	⅓ cup	370
Cantaloupe	¼ cup	341
Orange (navel)	1 medium	250
Strawberries	1 cup	247
Salt substitutes	1 tsp	
Morton lite salt		1500
Morton salt substitute		2800
No Salt		2500
No salt (seasoned)		1330

Hypertension, along with elevated cholesterol counts and cigarette smoking, is one of the Big Three risk factors for heart disease as well as for stroke. Start controlling your blood pressure with the lifestyle modifications I've discussed. See how well you do. For mild to moderate elevations, that should do the trick. For more severe cases of hypertension you may need to work with your doctor to find medication to bring it into the normal range. It's worth the effort. Your reward can be a longer, healthier life.

12
A Simple Proposal
for Weight Control

Americans are getting fatter and fatter. Well, not just Americans, but we're among the worst. Just take a stroll through Disneyland. In the 1980s, one in four of us was overweight. Statistics in 1998 revealed that number rose to one in three.

The weight problem isn't just a matter of cosmetics. Excessive weight increases the risk of heart disease, high blood pressure, and diabetes. Overweight men and women do not live as long as those who maintain a healthy weight. Fat kills.

Like jackals circling the weak, the diet industry has made millions on the misfortune of others. Infomercials on TV promise "amazing" weight loss with no exercise. Products abound. "Thermogenic" agents are said to burn fat. Others claim to block fat. Bunk. All the exaggerations are closely examined by corporate lawyers who keep their companies just within the letter of the law. And the laws governing the industry are lax, to say the least.

We'd all like to believe that by simply swallowing some magic pill we can continue to live sedentary, couch-potato existences while eating huge amounts of food. Yet typical expert advice of "eat less and exercise more" is simplistic.

And, since confession is good for the soul, I'll admit that the advice I provided back in the 1980s didn't do the trick. I wrote then that by cutting back on fat, you didn't need to worry about calories. Fat is the most dense source of calories, with 9 calories per gram, as compared with just 4 calories for carbohydrates and protein. Cut way back on fat, and the products that contain fat, and those pounds will melt away. Sounds good in theory, and for a while that approach actually worked.

In the mid- to late 1980s, there were practically no low-fat or nonfat foods on the market, so people who took my fat-cutting advice to heart would have to give up doughnuts, ice cream, crackers, and most desserts. Then the food industry saw a niche and quickly filled it. Suddenly we had fat-free everything.

Unfortunately, sugar filled in for the missing fat, and the calories per serving remained the same. Even worse, many felt empowered by those "fat-free" labels to consume unlimited amounts. A serving size became half the cake rather than a 1-inch slice. Instead of losing weight, these "dieters" gained more.

Yes, if one were to strictly limit fat intake while also avoiding the temptations of sugary treats, sticking with brussels sprouts and broccoli, one could, to use the promise of a best-selling book, "eat more, weigh less." Outside people in monasteries and convents, few seem able to do that.

You don't need another weight-loss book. You certainly don't need any of those "miracle" products touted in the infomercials or health food stores or by the multilevel-marketing companies. If you're really serious about losing those extra pounds once and for all, this chapter contains all the information you need. That's a promise.

TIME FOR A PERSONAL ANALYSIS

So what do *you* have to lose? Just a few pounds you picked up over the holidays or on vacation? Perhaps 10 to 20 pounds that have stubbornly hung on since you had the children? More? The truth is, even small amounts of excess weight have a negative effect on health. In a long-term study of tens of thousands of nurses, researchers saw that there was a linear scale in which obesity correlated with disease risk. The closer you can come to an ideal, healthy weight, the better.

What is a "healthy" weight? Sometimes the obvious manifestations are the most accurate. Does your belt have an increasing number of notches? Do clothes no longer fit? Does it seem that clothes designers are making "your" size smaller every year? Do you resist having your photo taken at family gatherings?

Healthy weight does not mean an unrealistic, impossible-to-attain figure. The ideal is not what we regularly see on magazine covers and television. A healthy weight is just that—*healthy*. A weight that is conducive to good health, not to landing a job as a runway fashion model. Ballerinas who smoke two packs of cigarettes a day, take laxatives, and induce vomiting to maintain a svelte figure are not healthy. They should not be role models for you or anyone else.

But if you were once comfortable in a size 8 dress or a 32-inch trouser and now are wearing a size 14 dress or a 38-inch slack, it's time to turn back the clock. And by doing so you'll also turn back the clock on your physiologic age.

Another, more scientific way to determine healthy body weight is to measure the percentage of your weight that is fat. Ironically, you can weigh practically the same as you did a few years ago and yet be more fat. Let me explain.

A football player at 6 feet tall and 220 pounds might be "overweight" according to weight scales, yet most of that weight may be solid muscle. Conversely, a slender girl who seldom if ever exercises may have excess fat and very little muscle tissue, even though her bathroom scales tell a happy tale.

The human body is composed of bone, muscle, and fat. Of those, only muscle can burn calories. Muscle tissue is the engine of the body. As one gets older and typically more sedentary, the percentage of muscle tissue shrinks, to be gradually replaced with fat. Sort of like a well-marbled piece of beef. Total weight may well remain the same for a while, but with less muscle burning those calories, fat tissue increases and weight gradually rises.

Two principal ways to determine body fat are being used today. The more accurate method is underwater weighing. The person to be weighed gets on a specially designed scale and is lowered into a pool of water. The buoyant fat does not register on the scale; only the bone and muscle get weighed. A simple calculation determines the percentage of body fat in relation to total body weight.

Not nearly as accurate, but a lot more convenient and adequate for many purposes, are skin fold measurements. A trained professional such as a registered dietitian uses calipers to measure the folds of skin at different sites on the body, principally the skin fold hanging from the underside of the arm at the triceps muscle. Unfortunately, recently introduced bathroom scales that claim to measure percentages of fat are not very accurate.

What fat percentages might one expect? A trained male athlete has between 5 and 13 percent body fat; female athletes measure in at 12 to 22 percent. For optimal health, men come in at 10 to 25 percent, and women should measure 18 to 30 percent fat. Obesity is determined as over 25 percent fat for men and over 30 percent for women.

Today health professionals rely on the body mass index (BMI) to assess healthy weight. This is a measure of body fat that corrects for height. It's determined by dividing weight in kilograms by the square of height in meters. More about that in a moment. The critical dividing line between healthy and unhealthy weight seems to be a BMI of 27. Even better is 25. Beyond that point, the risk of heart disease, diabetes, and hypertension climbs rapidly.

Here's how to determine your own BMI in the privacy of your own home. No calipers. No dunking in a pool of water. For practical purposes, we'll use pounds rather than kilograms and height in inches instead of meters. Just plug your own numbers into this equation:

$$BMI = \frac{703 \times \text{weight in pounds}}{\text{height in inches}^2}$$

Here's an example for a person who is 5 feet 9 inches (69 inches) weighing 162 pounds.

$$BMI = \frac{703 \times 162}{69 \times 69}$$

$$= \frac{113886}{4761}$$

$$= 24$$

With a BMI of 24, our example would be considered healthy by current National Heart Lung and Blood Institute guidelines. If he or she were to gain 7 pounds, however, the BMI would rise to 25, the cutoff point for being overweight. In the past, overweight was considered at 27 or greater BMI. That was before we knew how critical even small weight gains can be in undermining health. Those with a BMI of 30 or more are diagnosed as being clinically obese, requiring definite action to lose weight.

Table 10. **Body Mass Index (BMI)**

Height	Weight				
5 ft, 1 in.	127	132	137	143	158
5 ft, 2 in.	131	136	142	147	164
5 ft, 3 in.	135	141	146	152	169
5 ft, 4 in.	140	145	151	157	174
5 ft, 5 in.	144	150	156	162	180
5 ft, 6 in.	148	150	156	162	186
5 ft, 7 in.	153	159	166	172	191
5 ft, 8 in.	158	164	171	177	197
5 ft, 9 in.	162	169	176	182	203
5 ft, 10 in.	167	174	181	188	207
5 ft, 11 in.	172	179	186	193	215
6 ft	177	184	191	199	221
6 ft, 1 in.	182	189	197	204	227
BMI	24*	25**	26**	27**	30***

* healthy   **overweight   ***obese

Table 10 gives you an at-a-glance look at some sample BMI measures. Numbers are the same for both men and women. A BMI of 24 is considered healthy; 25 to 27 indicates overweight; 30 or more is obese.

SO WHAT'S THE ANSWER TO WEIGHT CONTROL?

Most of the weight loss books to hit the market, and often the bestseller list, are more nonsense than science. They cleverly begin with a tidbit of science, then make the leap to a nonscientific conclusion and go on to a nonsensical recommendation. Eating foods based on your blood type? Bunk. Combining foods in certain proportions? Witchcraft. But thanks to the First Amendment freedom of speech provision in the U.S. Constitution, people can publish anything they want.

Unless you've been living on a desert island, you know about all those recent books touting one form or another of low-carbohydrate diet. In truth, the *essence* of the low-carb approach is actually perfectly valid.

The low-carb diet can give you the satisfying weight loss you want in a reasonable amount of time and without feeling constantly deprived and hungry. But instead of having to read a whole book about this, all you need to know about this most efficient approach is right here in this chapter. No extra charge.

In this case I'm going to start with science and finish with science. It all began with the work of two world-renowned researchers, Drs. Bruce Bistrian and George Blackburn at Boston Deaconess Hospital. They noted that starvation diets, even when supervised in hospital settings, resulted in excessive muscle loss. In fact, those who refuse to eat as a form of political protest often die from heart failure owing to the loss of muscle tissue in this organ, long before they became ultrathin and skeletal in appearance.

The two doctors designed a diet that provided a small amount of fat, a large amount of high-quality protein, and a limited amount of carbohydrate. The logic behind this approach was simple. Fat is a concentrated source of calories, so it should be greatly restricted. Protein is essential to sparing muscle tissue, so it should be available. But why limit carbohydrates?

Severe carbohydrate restriction leads to a state of "ketosis" in which ketone bodies are produced and excreted in the urine. Ketosis serves two functions: First, one's appetite is greatly curtailed. Second, muscle tissue is spared since ketones are used by the body as a carbohydrate replacement, obviating the need to produce glucose from protein in a process called gluconeogenesis.

At first, this dietary approach was conducted only under strict medical supervision in a few major hospitals. Slowly its safety and effectiveness were recognized, and the details of the diet were spelled out in medical symposia and the literature.

Then the marketers, smelling money, stepped into the picture. First a physician sold a concoction said to duplicate the Blackburn-Bistrian diet. But the protein was of such poor quality that the body couldn't absorb it properly, and, very sadly, dozens of women died.

Then came the infamous moment when Oprah Winfrey told the world that by consuming only a special diet drink called Optifast she had lost a wagonload of fat and expected to keep it off permanently. That prediction did not come true. Oprah gained back the weight and swore she'd never go on another diet.

About that time, I was working as a consultant for a chain of weight loss clinics in the United States and Canada. Clients were supervised by nurses and followed a rather strict program of moderate exercise and a diet designed by a weight control authority at UCLA, Dr. Ernst Drenick.

Instead of a powder-based concoction or prepackaged frozen foods, clients ate a diet of natural foods they bought in their own supermarkets or restaurants. That diet was, in fact, very low in carbohydrates, even though it contained a number of vegetables and salads. After just a few days, the dieters felt they weren't very hungry and found the low-calorie food plan more than satisfying. Weight loss came quickly and clients were pleased with the way they looked in the mirror and the compliments they got.

Very importantly, that weight loss was maintained far better than in other programs. Why? Because the entire process involved a reeducation on eating habits.

But then came a diet that infuriated the medical and dietitian communities. It was the Dr. Atkins Diet Revolution. Dr. Atkins picked up on the notion that severely limiting carbohydrates resulted in a state of ketosis that killed appetite. And he attracted thousands of men and women with his promise that they could eat all the steaks, cheese, hamburgers, butter, and cream they wanted and still lose weight.

Critics were enraged. "Ketosis is dangerous and can destroy the kidneys," they said. "Avoiding nourishing foods will undermine health." "Eating all that fatty food makes you nauseated and you lose your appetite." Extreme criticism of what certainly is an extreme diet. But if one peels the layers of exaggeration from the underlying truths, we find an approach that offers weight loss success to even those who have failed and failed again in the past.

KOWALSKI'S CHANGE OF HEART

For quite a while, I straddled the fence between traditional "eat less, exercise more" and "low-carb" dietary plans. I felt that for most people, cutting back on fats would be enough to achieve weight control. And at the same time I worked with Dr. Calvin Ezrin, a world-renowned endocrinologist at Cedars-Sinai Medical Center in Los Angeles on a low-carb approach, primarily for diabetic patients with significant obesity.

Over the years since *The 8-Week Cholesterol Cure,* I have come to the conclusion that a sensible low-carbohydrate diet is the best regimen for weight loss, whether you have just a few extra pounds or a health-threatening excess. The emphasis is on the word *sensible.*

First and foremost, "low-carb" is not synonomous with "high-fat." Nor does it mean unlimited amounts of protein-rich steaks and chops. This is not the kind of "amazing" diet that will elicit either controversy or best-sellerdom with appearances on all the talk shows.

On the other hand, as a reward for some significant effort on your part, I can assure you of wonderfully satisfying success. Men can expect to lose about 4 pounds per week, while women will experience a weekly loss of about 3 pounds. After about three days of carbohydrate restriction, you won't be hungry. Many tell me it takes even less than three days. You'll be making some changes in food selection that will enable you to maintain your weight loss permanently.

Very importantly, this program is completely safe. I feel so strongly about that that I put both my wife and my 19-year-old daughter on the diet when they wanted to lose a few pounds. Both succeeded beautifully. Jenny was the envy of her teenaged friends, who wanted to know all about her "secrets." My family is precious to me, and I would never do anything to jeopardize their health.

Research at the famed Duke University, announced in July, 2002, found that a low-carbohydrate diet (less than 25 g/day) resulted in a weight loss of 10 percent of body weight over a six-month period in obese individuals. No limit was placed on fat or protein intake. Weight loss could have been quicker and more substantial if those calories had also been restricted by choosing low-fat meats and cheeses.

THE PROGRAM THAT WORKS

For starters, you want to enter a mild state of ketosis in which your body burns stored fats as energy. This results in ketone bodies in your urine, which you will monitor by way of Ketostix, available in any drugstore with no prescription needed.

You'll achieve ketosis by consuming no more than 40 grams of carbohydrates a day. I'll spell out carbohydrate contents of foods shortly, but suffice it to say that 40 grams is not very much. In fact, at the very beginning—for the first few days at least—you might want to "jump on the ketosis express" by completely avoiding all carbohydrates, or as much as possible. That means no bread, no rice, no pasta, no dairy foods, no foods that list carbohydrates on the nutrition label.

After three days, put a Ketostix strip into your urine stream. It should change color—becoming pink to light purple—indicating a mild state of ketosis. Compare your strip to the color code on the Ketostix bottle. There is no benefit to a deeper color change. Just the slightest bit of ketosis is all it takes to diminish appetite and start burning that stored fat.

During those early days, concentrate on high-protein foods that are also low in fat. Remember, you're burning your stored fat. You don't need any additional fat, and eating more just slows down the weight loss process. Good choices would include lean meats, fish, shellfish, eggs and egg substitutes, chicken and beef broths, and sausages. Be sure to read the labels of processed meats; many contain added carbohydrates, you'll be surprised to find.

During the entire weight loss period, you'll just have to bite the bullet when it comes to desserts. Sugar is a big culprit in America's collective weight problem, and you'll want to avoid it at all costs. Satisfy your need for something sweet with sugar-free popsicles, sugar-free Jell-O, and sugar-free toppings such as D-Zerta.

Probably the biggest difference in my approach to the low-carb diet comes down to a reeducation of your eating habits. This is the time to learn portion control. Most people have no idea how much they're actually eating; it's no surprise they gain weight.

Speaking of not knowing what one is actually eating, and how much, the first thing you'll want to do is *start keeping a journal*. Jot down everything you eat and drink, and in what quantity. This is especially important on a low-carb diet, since you'll want to note exactly how many carbs you're taking in from this food or that. Remember, no more than 40 grams per day. Strive to keep the carb grams in the mid-30s range.

What about Alcoholic Beverages?

Some have no carbs at all, including dry white or red wines and spirits such as gin, scotch, and vodka. Others, notably beer and sweet drinks, are loaded with carbs. The noncarb alcoholic beverages will not take you out of ketosis. However, all alcohol packs calories. Perhaps most important, a drink or two can loosen inhibitions and lead you to indulge in foods you'd otherwise avoid. During the initial weight loss period you're better off completely abstaining from alcohol.

Snacking Is a Good Thing on a Low-Carb Diet

Studies have shown time and again that those who eat many little meals throughout the day, rather than gorging on just one or two large ones, tend to maintain ideal weight. Learning to plan and enjoy healthy low-carb snacks daily is part of your reeducation. Some good ideas might include a cup of broth, a hard-cooked egg, a small piece of fruit, some vegetable sticks, or a slice of low-fat sausage.

Don't Forget to Exercise Daily

It doesn't have to be much, but keep active now and for the rest of your life. Instead of that coffee and doughnut during your morning and afternoon breaks, take a 10- or 15-minute walk. Take the stairs rather than the elevator. Park your car at the farthest point in the lot. Plan physical activity such as bike riding or a weekend hike in the woods for your leisure time. Exercise is an indispensable part of weight control.

FOODS FOR YOUR LOW-CARB DIET

You're going to lose weight on a low-carb diet even if you don't restrict your calories. But you won't lose that weight as quickly. Don't you want to achieve your goal as soon as possible? And by carefully planning portions of this food and that, you'll be well on your way to permanent weight maintenance.

Don't be too shocked by this, but I'd like you to limit yourself to about 850 calories a day. Men can do well with another 150 calories—1000 calories total.

Won't you be hungry? In a word, no. Ketosis will take care of the hunger very nicely. You might want more food only because you're used to eating more, so it's more a psychological rather than a physiological need. Moreover, you'll be burning that stored fat that you want to get rid of once and for all. By limiting total calories and remaining in ketosis, you'll free about 1000 calories from stored fat daily. That means your body will actually be "fed" 1850 to 2000 calories daily. More than enough!

So what should you eat and what should you avoid? Certainly

stay away from all forms of sugar. Just one or two pieces of candy can take you out of ketosis. And once you're out, it's far more difficult to get back into that wonderful, appetite-suppressing state. You'll also want to avoid all starchy foods during your weight loss period. These include breads, cereals, rice, pasta, beans and lentils, and certain vegetables—corn, lima beans, peas, potatoes, squash, and yams.

While fruits provide a wonderful array of nutrients and antioxidants, you'll want to limit both fruits and fruit juices while you're in ketosis. One serving of fruit—a small apple, a medium banana, ½ cup of fruit cocktail, two plums, ½ cup of juice—averages 15 grams of carbohydrate. This is the time to start working on portion control: have just a little bit now and then.

Most dairy foods—milk, yogurt, cottage cheese—have quite a lot of carbohydrate. Although they are excellent sources of calcium and other nutrients, avoid milk products during weight loss. Supplement your diet with calcium.

Fish, shellfish, lean meats of all sorts, and poultry have no carbohydrates at all. Enjoy a reasonable serving, about 4 to 6 ounces, three times daily.

Although fats and oils contain no carbohydrate whatever, they all provide 12 to 15 grams of fat and a lot of calories per tablespoon. Use them sparingly during weight loss.

This is a great time to increase your daily intake of salads and vegetables. Enjoy all the spinach, romaine, endive, lettuce, escarole, cabbage, celery, cucumber, mushrooms, radishes, and peppers you wish. Have them steamed or lightly sautéed as a side dish for your meals. Prepare them as salads with vinaigrette dressings; read the labels of commercial products to check for added carbs. Make a variety of hot soups, using broths as a base.

As beverages, go for lots and lots of water every day, along with diet sodas, coffee and tea, sugar-free cocoa, and bouillon. A squeeze of lemon or lime makes a glass of club soda a festive drink, served with lots of ice in nice goblet.

Instead of sugar, use artificial sweeteners including NutraSweet (Equal), Sugar Twin, or others.

What might a typical day's meal plan look like? For breakfast, one egg, any style, a cup of beef bouillon, and a small serving of fruit or juice, perhaps a 3-ounce glass of juice or a ¼ cup of fruit cocktail, or half an orange. Lunch might be a piece of chicken or fish, about 4 to 5 ounces, along with a salad and vinaigrette dressing and perhaps sugar-free gelatin for dessert. An afternoon snack might consist of a slice of sausage and a few grapes. Dinner will typically be another protein dish, a small serving of vegetable such as asparagus or broccoli, a nice big salad or cup of soup, and a sugar-free dessert. Don't forget to drink lots of fluids throughout the day.

Can you eat more than these allowances? Can you have a glass of wine or a cocktail? How about some olive oil on that salad? Sure, but all these add calories and slow down the process of weight loss.

SOME TRICKS TO ENSURE SUCCESS

- *Get all the support you can.* Tell the "whole world" that you've decided to improve your health and happiness by losing those extra pounds. Ask a friend to go on the diet with you for mutual support. Make it an adventure!
- *Treat yourself.* Even though you won't be hungry, thanks to the ketosis, you'll be giving up one of life's greatest pleasures: eating. This is the time to replace that pleasure with treats for yourself. Perhaps a daily bubble bath with candles burning and soft music playing. Maybe 30 minutes a day set aside to read a novel. A weekly manicure or pedicure or a bottle of perfume purchased with the food money you've saved.
- *Make some lifestyle changes.* Many people become preoccupied with food: shopping, planning, preparation, going to restaurants. Spend some of that time doing other things. Take in more movies. Go shoot a game of pool. Attend a concert or lecture. Take a computer class.
- *Behavior modification really works.* Some of these ideas may seem strange or quaint, but researchers have demonstrated time and again that they get the job done. The whole thing is to change the patterns you normally follow regarding food. Don't eat in front of the TV or while reading; in doing so, you lose track of the amount of food you eat. Eat in one designated location; for example, don't eat in bed or in the living room. Most people don't eat anything more after they've brushed their teeth for the evening; do that brushing early in the evening rather than closer to bedtime. Avoid situations you normally associate with eating; substitute them with other activities where food is out of the picture, such as a trip to the museum.
- *Follow the tried and true.* Some of the old bits of advice still hold true. Put your meals on smaller plates so they look fuller. Eat more slowly, savoring every mouthful. Put the fork down between bites. Drink a big glass of water a few minutes before each meal. Wear an article of clothing that's too small now, but into which you'll fit easily when you've lost those pounds.

TWO STEPS TO PERMANENT WEIGHT CONTROL

How many times have you lost weight only to gain it all back and more? You don't want that to happen again, and it really doesn't have to.

Once you've reached the weight you wanted—and once again, it's important to go all the way to that healthy weight and not stop short of your goal—you've finished only the first step toward permanent weight control. Unfortunately, most of the diets people read about and follow end when the weight is lost. People breathe a sigh of relief, buy some new clothes, and then go right back to the bad eating habits that led to the weight problem in the first place.

This time it's going to be different. The next step is a period of *stabilization*. During this time, you very gradually add back some foods you've either eliminated or restricted. You'll want to find out, in a very structured, deliberate way, just how much food you can consume now without either losing more weight or gaining any of those pounds back. Begin the first day of stabilization by adding just one slice of toast with your morning breakfast. Do that for a few days and check your weight. No problem? Terrific. Now add another serving of vegetables to your evening dinner.

Take your time with this. Add one little bit of food at a time. Consult the scales regularly. Did you gain a pound? Ease back for the next couple of days. Eventually you'll know exactly how much food in general, and how much carbohydrate in particular, you can have to maintain that healthy weight.

Now it's finally time to enter the period of *maintenance*. To paraphrase, this is the first day of the rest of your new, healthy, slender life. Thousands of men and women have done it before you, and there's no reason in the world you won't succeed.

During the weight loss and stabilization periods, you've learned a great deal about your body. You're now more conscious of the foods you select and eat. You are regularly engaging in physical activity, hopefully a minimum of 30 minutes every day. You know the foods that can put you back into a weight gain mode. Those, of course, are the foods high in carbohydrates.

Simply, you'll want to limit carbohydrates, especially the sugars, permanently. Choose the ones that have some nutritional benefits along with the carbs and calories. Beans, for example, are packed with soluble fiber that helps control cholesterol. Fruits are loaded with vitamins and antioxidants. Breads, pastas, rice, desserts, potatoes, and other starchy foods have very little to offer nutritionally. Sure, the whole-grain varieties are the exception, but let's face it, most people don't eat them. So as much as it is possible for you to do so, avoid those starchy foods forever.

If a person who had some weight to lose did nothing more than eliminate the empty-calorie, nutrient-poor starchy carbohydrate foods such as breads and pasta and cakes and cookies, he or she would gradually lose a great deal of weight without ever following a structured diet!

If you learn nothing else from this chapter, burn that last paragraph into your mind and keep it there for the rest of your life.

In a perfect world, every single one of my readers would follow the advice of this chapter, lose those extra pounds, and never gain the weight back. But this is the real world and people do slip. Perhaps you'll gain 5 pounds or so on vacation or during the holidays. All is not lost. But don't lose any time—get back on the straight and narrow. Perhaps you'll be able to shed those reappearing pounds simply by cutting back on starchy foods. But a more efficient approach would be to go back to square one by starting the weight loss process all over again and entering ketosis and eliminating most carbohydrates—once again limiting yourself to no more than 40 grams daily. This time it won't take as long to get back to where you want to be.

The rewards of achieving a healthy goal weight are enormous. Your cholesterol, triglycerides, and blood pressure will come down. You'll sleep better and awake energized and refreshed. You'll feel better about yourself. It's *definitely* worth the effort.

13

The Heart of Your Emotions

A man gets angry on the job; an hour later he suffers a heart attack. A woman tends to have the "blues" more often than not; unlike her more upbeat peers, she does not recover from her bypass surgery. Coincidences? Not too many years ago, doctors dismissed the mind-body connection as unfounded. Today we have solid research to show the heart has a mind of its own.

In a very real way, one can compare the influence of the emotions on heart disease with the effect of elevated cholesterol. When the latter link was first spotted in the 1960s and 1970s, many physicians doubted the connection. My editor even questioned why I wanted a chapter on stress in *The 8-Week Cholesterol Cure*. I had to fight for it.

As the research data have accumulated over the years, most physicians now recognize negative emotions as risk factors for heart disease. Although papers are routinely delivered at meetings of the American Heart Association, that organization has not officially designated stress, depression, and other negative emotions as risk factors to the same degree as they have with, say, cholesterol or high blood pressure.

That's largely because emotional states are difficult to measure in a discrete manner. Doctors like to have numbers to measure and treat patients—do a test, find an elevated number, prescribe a drug, end of problem. I'm sure that someday soon that situation will change.

But right now, deep down inside, you know that emotions have an effect on your heart. Even little kids experience skipped beats in scary situations. Our hearts pound when we get angry or frustrated and "sink" when we are seriously disappointed. Our blood pressure rises with the anxiety of a physician's examination—it's called "white-coat hypertension."

When do most heart attacks occur? On Monday mornings at the

beginning of the stressful week. Authorities think this is not a coincidence, and research data bear them out. Ironically, the winter holidays bring out a cluster of heart-related deaths. Many think it is the stress of planning, or the depression of being alone, or the unattainability of the perfect Norman Rockwell holiday experience.

In the early 1970s, doctors coined the term "type A personality" to decribe those most likely to have heart disease. Such individuals were said to be driven, time-oriented workaholics. Nice theory, but it collided with the fact that many people really loved that lifestyle and reveled in their successful careers. If all type A's died of heart attacks, we'd have no top businesspeople, doctors, entertainment executives, or politicians.

The emotions that kill are more subtle. Anger and hostility, hopelessness, frustration and depression, even everyday stress and strain and sadness. Combine two or more types of negative emotions and the effect is cumulative. Add those to other risk factors, including high blood pressure, diabetes, and elevated cholesterol counts, and the impact can be deadly.

I've known about how stress kills for years, well before any research was being done. Case in point: my own father. Dad was a man who loved his wife every day of his marriage, adored his children, and reveled in his career as a respected neighborhood pharmacist. His hypertension was being medically treated, he remained physically fit and slender, didn't smoke, and drank very little.

Then a tragic occurrence at his place of work changed his life. He came to hate going to work but felt duty-bound to his customers. The effects were dramatic and Dad's hypertension went out of control. He looked haggard and was always tired. Within a few months, my father was dead of a massive heart attack, preceded, we now believe, by a couple of small strokes. That was in 1969. He was only 57 years old.

Fast forward to 1978. In addition to a family history, an elevated cholesterol level, cigarette smoking, and lack of exercise, I encountered a situation that put me into a myriad of negative emotions. Twenty-four hours a day, seven days a week, I felt angry, depressed, and hopeless—a long story not worth telling, but within a few months, at 35, I suffered a heart attack.

Jump to 1995. My brother had experienced a business failure that brought him from a point of early prosperity to near bankruptcy. He went from a happy-go-lucky sort to a cigarette-smoking, nail-biting, stressed-out mess. His heart attack hit about a year later. Tom was 49. Fortunately, he survived.

Those are what the doctors like to call "anecdotal" stories, not scientific evidence of any link betweeen heart disease and our emotional states. But today we have the kind of hard-nosed, scientifically controlled research data that no one can deny. Here is a small sampling.

THE IRONCLAD CASE FOR
THE MIND-BODY-HEART CONNECTION

Anger-Prone People Are More Likely to Have Heart Attacks

- A person who is most prone to anger is about three times more likely to have a heart attack or suffer sudden cardiac death than someone who is the least hotheaded. Those who scored as being somewhat moderate in their anger were still 35 percent more likely to experience a coronary event. These findings, coming from the University of North Carolina in May 2000, held true even after accounting for other risk factors, including smoking, diabetes, cholesterol, and overweight. The study lasted six years. At the beginning, no one had any sign of heart disease. By the end, of a total of nearly 13,000 men and women, 256 individuals had heart attacks. They were the ones who had previously tested as being the most anger prone.

- The movie *Grumpy Old Men* was a comedy, but the reality is that older men who scored highest in anger on a personality test were three times more likely to suffer a heart attack in a seven-year study than calmer individuals. In 1997, a Harvard Medical School investigation found a direct relationship between anger and heart disease.

- In a 1995 study done in cooperation with 55 different medical centers in the United States, doctors found that the deadly potential of anger can strike quickly. The risk of having a heart attack among more than 1600 patients, both men and women, was 2.3 times as great in the first two hours after an anger outburst, as compared with those who had not experienced anger prior to their coronary events.

Depression Can Be a Real Heartbreaker

- From 1948 to 1995, medical students at Johns Hopkins University were surveyed in a study to determine the precursors of heart disease. Of nearly 1200 men, 12 percent had clinical depression beginning on average at age 46. There were no differences in other coronary risk factors between the depressed and nondepressed subjects in the study. But depressed individuals were twice as likely to develop coronary heart disease, suffer a heart attack, or have a sudden cardiac death. This was the first dramatic proof that depression could be a factor in *developing* heart disease.

■ Depression has also been shown to be a risk factor for increased mortality following a heart attack. British researchers tracked more than 5600 patients, both men and women. During the study, 188 men and 139 women were diagnosed as having heart disease or heart attack. Compared with others who also had accompanying risk factors such as smoking and high blood pressure, those suffering with depression were three times more likely to succumb to heart disease.

■ Depression need not be severe to have adverse effects on the heart. That was demonstrated in a 1996 study, also at Johns Hopkins, with those who had a history of periodic bouts of depression defined as two weeks of sadness. They experienced slightly more than twice the likelihood of having a heart attack. Those with a major depressive episode were 4.5 times more likely to have a heart attack than those not suffering from depression.

■ Similar results have been noted by researchers around the world. Danish doctors wrote in 1996 that depression is a risk factor for heart disease that, like other risk factors, is linear in its effects. That is to say, the worse the depression, the worse the effects on the heart. But at either end of the depression scale, impact on the heart is very real. The headline of the news release put out on the research by the American Heart Association read "Being Chronically 'Blue' Raises Risk of Heart Attack."

■ Depression also plays a role in stroke risk. Scientists from the National Center for Health Statistics analyzed data from a 16-year study. They found that major depression raised the risk of having a stroke about as much as did a 40-point increase in systolic blood pressure (the top number). Severe depressive symptoms created an even greater risk than did other risk factors, including smoking, obesity, diabetes, and elevated cholesterol.

■ The term "depression" includes many emotional feelings, including that of hopelessness. As reported in the February

2000 issue of the journal *Hypertension,* feelings of hopelessness lead to the development of high blood pressure. That, in turn, increases the probability of future heart disease.

SUFFERING FROM STRESS
PUTS YOUR HEART IN A MESS

I've communicated by mail and spoken with literally thousands of men and women since first publishing my book back in 1987. The vast majority put the real blame for their heart attacks, bypass surgeries, and other events on stress. Sure, they would admit, their diets hadn't been the best and their lifestyles weren't the healthiest but the ultimate culprit, they said and deeply believed, was stress.

This is not a thing to be taken lightly as too many doctors still do. Stress ranks right up there with cholesterol, high blood pressure, and the other biggies. It would be foolish to continue to smoke with the cavalier attitude that "I've dealt with the other risk factors, isn't that enough?" Similarly, why dismiss stress or ignore it?

Stress can not only contribute to the development of heart disease, it can also act as the precipitating factor for a heart attack or stroke. Again, we now have the research to back this up.

Whether stress is chronic and unrelenting or acute and sudden, the effects can be deadly. I very well remember the day in January 1994 when a big earthquake struck the Los Angeles area. Fortunately for us, the event was simply startling and we suffered no significant damage. But those closer to the epicenter did not fare as well. The number of sudden cardiac deaths jumped dramatically, from an average of fewer than 5 per typical day the previous week to 24 the day of the earthquake.

Interestingly, the incidence of sudden cardiac death the week after the quake dropped to a low 2.7 on average per day. Why? Apparently those who had died the week before died prematurely, "shocked" into the heart attack that might have waited until later had it not been for the precipitating factor.

Researchers had previously shown that other stressful situations—episodes of anger, heavy physical or emotional exertion, fear, divorce, bankruptcy—can trigger cardiac events. Although the exact mechanism by which this happens is not known, most doctors now believe it's a matter of disrupting a soft, vulnerable plaque in the coronary arteries, thus spilling the gooey contents into the blood and forming a big clot that blocks off blood flow to the heart muscle. We also know that stress results in production of chemicals in the body, including adrenaline and cortisol, which speed up heart rate and increase blood pressure.

A Finnish study with 901 men found that those with the most extreme blood pressure responses to a mental stress test had the thickest blockages from atherosclerosis in the carotid arteries, which convey blood to the brain. That was especially true for men under 55 years of age. Dr. Thomas Kamarck of the University of Pittsburgh, who was the study's lead author in the journal *Circulation,* said that just like elevated cholesterol, mental stress over time may injure blood vessels and promote atherosclerosis in those individuals who are particularly susceptible to emotional swings.

Stress takes many different forms. It certainly need not be as dramatic as the fear from the earthquake or the shock of financial ruin. Some individuals simply live with a sense of hopelessness, a feeling that things are not going to get better. A four-year study of nearly 1000 middle-aged men linked such hopelessness to faster progression of heart disease. Those who had indicated by way of tests that they had given up hope in their lives had a 20 percent greater increase in the atherosclerosis process, diagnosed by way of ultrasound, compared to their more optimistic peers.

A major study published in the *Journal of the American Medical Association* concluded that mental stress during daily life, including feelings of tension, frustration, and sadness, can more than double the risk of interrupting blood flow to the heart. When the heart receives inadequate blood and oxygen through the coronary arteries, one may experience the chest pains known as angina. And in extreme cases, the result could be a heart attack.

For those who have already had a heart attack, stress can increase their chances of suffering another one. Belgian researchers found that negative, insecure, and anxious patients were three times as likely to have another heart attack. According to Dr. Redford Williams at Duke University, people with a lot of negative emotions who tend to keep those feelings bottled up are more likely to have a poor outcome than other patients.

Some doctors are now thinking that patients should be given an emotional stress test in addition to the standard physical stress test typically done on a treadmill. Studies have shown that when challenged to do, say, a mentally taxing arithmetic problem, patients can experience the same sort of interrupted flow of blood to the heart as they get through physical activity.

Okay, you've had an extremely stressful day. You've been angry at business associates, and frustrated about the turn of events. At dinner you console yourself with a particularly large, rich dinner. Bad choice. It turns out that both stress and those big, fatty meals lead to increased levels of the fats known as triglycerides in the blood. Combining the two can be a deadly recipe, with blood fats so thick that a heart attack can occur.

SO WHAT CAN YOU DO ABOUT IT?

Stress is like the weather: Everybody talks about it, but few do anything about it. I certainly didn't spell out all the scary studies in this chapter simply to frighten you. Like elevated cholesterol, negative emotional states can increase your risk of heart disease and perhaps even a heart attack. And as with cholesterol, you can take the needed steps to reduce or eliminate this risk factor. Right now you just may be thinking, "Well, that's easy for you to say. You don't know how bad my situation really is." The fact is, everyone experiences stress and other emotional feelings. The real risk relates to how you deal with that stress and those feelings. You may not be able to stop the rain, but you sure can open your umbrella.

Granted, an umbrella will keep you dry in a rainstorm, but can stress-buster techniques really make a difference in heart health? In a word, yes. The *Journal of the American Medical Association* published a review article in April 2000 of studies dealing with stress and its treatment. In 20 controlled trials, for example, that evaluated the impact of psychosocial treatments for reducing stress-related factors, those getting the treatment fared far better than those who did not. Heart rate, blood pressure, and cholesterol levels fell. Psychological outlook improved and there was a lesser incidence of cardiac events, from chest pains to heart attacks to cardiac deaths.

The first step in reducing the risk of mental stress on your heart is to become aware of the stress in your own life, how much it affects you, and what you're doing about it. Most depressed and severely stressed men and women never get the help they need because they never ask for it. Sadly, not all doctors are knowledgeable about the mind-body-heart connection. They may ask about your smoking and eating habits but not about how you're feeling mentally. It's up to you to bring up your problems with your doctor. Once you do, you'll find that he or she will probably be quite open to the discussion and offer some suggestions to help you cope.

No matter how bad things may appear to be right now, there are a number of approaches to deal with your mental outlook. They range from self-help approaches to a variety of medications to formal psychological counseling. Let's work our way up through them.

It pays to be optimistic. We know from studies that pessimists die from heart disease far more than optimists. Pessimists are not only more likely to develop CHD, but they are also less likely to survive a heart attack when it happens. Some people are born optimists, always viewing the glass as half full. But you can choose to become more optimistic, and that's a good thing.

The half-full or half-empty glass analogy is the ultimate when it comes to learning to be more optimistic. Start in the morning as soon as you wake up. Congratulations! Why? Because you *did* wake up! You're about to have another day of life on this planet. And considering the alternative, that's a very good thing.

As you drive to work, instead of envying the Cadillacs and Mercedes, notice how many commuters have cars far more beat up and older than yours. If someone cuts you off in traffic, mentally conjure up a scenario in which your lifestyle is far better than his. Yes, the lousy so-and-so cut you off, but perhaps he has a shrew for a wife or is suffering from horrible back pain. Can't find a place to park close to the building? Great opportunity to get some exercise.

Take the old saying "Count your blessings" a step further by actually taking out a piece of paper and listing all the good things in your life. In another column, note the things you really like to do but never get around to doing. Maybe it's going to a movie or hitting a bucket of golf balls on the driving range or getting a massage or facial. Then make a point of actually scheduling those things. For example, why not plan to stop at the practice range to work on your golf swing on the way home from work? Maybe just for 15 minutes—be nice to yourself.

Balance that accounting ledger by also listing the bad things in your life. Almost surely, the good things will form a larger, longer column than the bad. But then examine that column and ask yourself what you might do to improve a particular situation. As another example, if you really, really *hate* that rush-hour traffic on the way home from work every day (as my wife does, having to battle the LA commute), why not join a gym near work and take a swim. By the time you're finished, traffic will have eased up.

An Australian study has shown us that it's not the stress one encounters on the job that's a killer, it's the way one deals with that stress. Subjects were workers in a tax office, definitely a stressful environment. Some responded by drinking, eating, and smoking more.

Their blood pressures went up. Others coped by turning to humor, hobbies, the support of friends, and exercise or other relaxation techniques. They had much better blood pressure scores. A note to the guys: Women did a lot better job of coping with stress in positive rather than negative ways.

A few little tips to cultivating optimism: if something goes wrong, don't always blame yourself. Carry in your wallet a few pictures of the people, places, and things that make you happy. When things turn nasty, whip out those photos and smile. Every time you find something wrong with yourself, bring to mind the traits others admire in you.

Want some positive feedback from others? Start giving it out. Compliment people on a new hairstyle or clothing. Give them an "attaboy" for a job well done. Simply smile at someone walking down the hall. It turns out that the muscles that control a frown in your face are hot-wired to the brain, which spews out stress hormones. It's nature's way of getting you ready for fight or flight. Conversely, when your facial muscles form a smile, the brain perceives that all is well and floods the bloodstream with calming neurotransmitters. If you actively smile during times when you would normally be frowning or worse, your brain sends out calming chemicals rather than hostile ones. It works that way even when you don't feel like smiling. Just do it. Sounds silly, and perhaps even preposterous, but it really does work.

Feeling all alone in life? Those who participate in support groups tend to be far healthier than those who go it on their own. For those recovering from heart attacks and bypass surgery, for example, the Mended Hearts group, based in Dallas, brings together folks in your situation. Call for local chapters in your area or try the national office at 214-706-1442. Join a church group or volunteer to do something for others like working at a homeless shelter. As the proverb goes, "Bread on the waters."

How would you like someone who would love you unconditionally? Someone who would run up to you when you came home, eager for your affection, who would want to be with you practically all the time, never finding fault, and always looking at you with adoring eyes. You need a pet!

No, this is not a joke. We have tons of data showing how having a pet vastly improves emotional health and actually protects against heart disease. As just one example, doctors at the State University of New York in Buffalo worked with 48 male and female stockbrokers who were using medication to control their hypertension. Those who owned a pet experienced half the increase in blood pressure under stress as those who did not. Both dogs and cats had similar calming effects during times of particular stress.

Tai chi—a slow, relaxed physical activity program originated in ancient China—lowered blood pressure in older adults nearly as much as moderate-intensity aerobic exercise. That was the finding of Johns Hopkins researchers. Ironically, the doctors expected the opposite. They didn't think tai chi would have much impact since it seems like so little effort is involved. I guess when something lasts literally for centuries, there must be something to it. If you're interested in trying it out, start with a call to your local YMCA or health club to find out about classes.

Another approach along similar lines is yoga. This has nothing to do with spiritualism or Eastern religions. Yoga is a discipline of stretching poses that improve flexibility, contribute to strength, and calm the mind and body. Yoga classes might be a lot easier to find than tai chi. You can even do yoga at home with a videotape, but you'll miss out on the distinct benefits of group participation.

Be nice to yourself. What have you done for others lately? You can probably rattle off a list a mile long with all sorts of things you do for your spouse and childen and family and friends, contributions to charity, work beyond the call of duty, volunteer work, and so on. But what have you done for yourself? If you're like most people, you've put yourself last on the priority list. It's time to change that.

This is not to say you should be doing self-destructive things like smoking, drinking excessively, staring at the TV while eating quantities of fat-laden foods. These really won't make you feel better. And they will hasten the development of heart disease.

Here's a wonderful way to "think" yourself into a good mood. It's called cognitive therapy and is something I've relied on heavily for years since I first learned about this approach to better mental health. Simply enough, the concept is that emotional problems are caused by looking at things the wrong way. In cognitive therapy, one learns to think differently.

This is not psychobabble. The therapeutic approach was first developed to offer a short-term treatment for depression. It appealed to those who could not or would not submit to months of clinical sessions. Today, cognitive therapy has been proved effective for dealing with anxiety, chronic fatigue, plain old garden-variety "blues," and daily stress. While professional counselors are available if necessary, cognitive therapy can be undertaken by the individual. You'll find a number of books on the subject in libraries and bookstores. Or visit the Academy of Cognitive Therapy on the Web at www.acadamofct.org. Or send a self-addressed stamped, business-sized envelope to the academy at One Belmont Avenue, Suite 700, Bala Cynwyd, PA 19004.

In the meantime, here are a few pointers on how to think more positively about your life:

- Give yourself credit for your accomplishments. Don't write them off as simply luck.
- Recognize the fact that others find many admirable traits in you. Be proud of those traits.
- Start thinking that you'll succeed rather than assuming you will fail. It will be a self-fulfilling prophecy.
- View your situation objectively as though it were the life of someone else and offer advice to that "other" person.
- Think of negative thoughts going through your head as static on the radio. "Turn" to a different station with a better program.
- Actively bring back memories of particularly happy times and places. Learn to visualize those past pleasures, and then use them to replace negative thoughts when they occur.
- Turn the simple act of breathing into an award-winning performance. Concentrate on breathing refreshing air in, filling your lungs to the absolute limit. Hold that breath for several seconds. Then gradually exhale, as though a balloon was being deflated. Do that for a few minutes several times daily. You'll get so good at it that you'll look forward to your conscious-breathing breaks as minivacations. During times of stress, turn to your deep breathing rather than focusing on the negatives in your life at the moment.
- Learn to spend more time in the moment rather than thinking about the past or the future. Deferred gratification is a good thing when it comes to saving money for retirement or taking courses that can lead to a job promotion. But don't let the present get away. As has been said many times in many ways, life is not a dress rehearsal. This is it. There's no second time around. Enjoy. Take your pleasures as often as possible, whether it's a little thing like stopping the car to actually look at a "scenic vista" or something bigger, such as dinner with family or friends.

WHEN YOU CAN'T GO IT ON YOUR OWN

Everyone can profit from these suggestions, but there are times that call for something beyond a few self-help tips. There are a lot of things you can do to help yourself prevent heart disease, but sometimes you need medical or even surgical assistance. Would you refuse help from a doctor trying to save your life during a heart attack? Would you refuse to take a prescription drug to control hypertension or cardiac arrhythmia? Probably not. Nor should you refuse the professional assistance of a trained psychological counselor if your troubles get too big for one person to handle. We know that severe depression can kill just as certainly as elevated cholesterol levels. Ask your doctor for a referral.

Your doctor might also see fit to prescribe a medication to help you cope. Maybe just a little something to help you get a better night's rest. Since we know that stresses can precipitate heart attacks, perhaps a prescription for an antihypersensitive medication such as a beta-blocker could lower both your heart rate and your blood pressure.

Taking that aspirin tablet each day might also protect you from your emotions. Doctors at the National Heart, Lung and Blood Institute found that daily aspirin can reduce the risk generated by outbursts of anger. Studying more than 1600 men and women, they learned that the overall "relative risk" of heart attack during the two hours after an episode of anger was 2.3 times higher than among those who were not angry. But among regular aspirin users, the relative risk was only 1.4: that's about half that in those who didn't use aspirin and not much higher than someone who had not been angry, whose relative risk would be 1.0. Now, don't use this as an excuse to continue to fly off the handle. But it's nice to know the buffer is there.

By now just about everyone knows about Prozac and the other medications that calm and soothe by increasing the serotonin levels in the brain. Some have profusely praised Prozac and some have damned it. Reality probably lies somewhere in between. For those with a significant problem with depression, Prozac can be a lifesaver.

If you definitely prefer to avoid prescription drugs, you might consider using St. John's wort. This herbal preparation is commonly used in Europe, especially in Germany where doctors prescribe it more often than Prozac. The German commission that regulates herbs and their usage in that country suggests 2 to 4 grams daily. Do *not* combine this herb with prescribed antidepressive drugs.

Another herbal remedy is the plant extract valerian, which can help you get the good night's sleep you need to better prepare you for the next day's stresses and strains. Valerian has been around for decades, and its safety and efficacy have been well documented. Again the herb is widely used in Europe. The German commission recommends 2 to 3 grams of the powdered root or extract, or up to 1 teaspoon of the tincture. Do not combine with sedatives or other sleeping pills.

ADDITIONAL BENEFITS OF STRESS MANAGEMENT

I'm confident that one day fairly soon the American Heart Association will formally designate stress and other emotional distress as risk factors for heart disease, right up there with hypertension, diabetes, and high cholesterol. As with those other factors, negative emotional states can be successfully treated and controlled. But while you might not feel any better from having a lowered blood pressure or cholesterol level, you'll enjoy life a whole lot more when depression, stress, anxiety, and other emotional burdens are lifted. What you'll have is a healthy, *happy* heart!

14
Healthy Surfing in Cyberspace

I must confess that I'm not much of a computer person. But the Internet does offer a universe of information. Unfortunately, however, you can't always trust what you find on a Web site, or in a chat room, or on a bulletin board. In fact, a lot of the content posted is loaded with quackery and is often meant to sell worthless products.

Separating the wheat from the chaff can be difficult if not impossible for the average person. Making a value judgment about a Web site is rather similar to judging the value of a print journal. Who publishes it? Does the group stand to profit from sales of products or services discussed? Has the material been reviewed by professionals in the field with no vested interest?

With these things in mind, combined with my experience in health communications for more than three decades, I have put together a listing of Web sites I think you'll find both informative and accurate. I'm sure that after surfing through them, many of these sites will wind up in your "favorites" file.

GENERAL NUTRITION AND HEALTH INFORMATION

International Food Information Council Foundation:
www.ifcinfo.health.org

Tufts University Nutrition Navigator:
www.navigator.tufts.edu

Dr. Koop's Community
www.drkoop.com

U.S. Federal Government/National Institutes of Health
www.nih.gov/health

Mayo Clinic
www.medhealth.org

Medscape (Service of CBS News)
www.medscape.com

American Medical Association
www.ama-assn.org/consumer.htm

FOOD SAFETY

The U.S. Federal Government/Department of Agriculture
www.foodsafety.gov

HERBAL REMEDIES AND ALTERNATIVE MEDICINE

Medical Herbalism Journal
www.medherb.com

Alternative Health News Online
www.altmedicine.com

Andrew Weil, M.D.
www.drweil.com

Natural Medicines Comprehensive Database Web Page
www.naturaldatabase.com

DIETARY SUPPLEMENTS: QUALITY AND SAFETY

Consumer Lab
www.consumerlab.com

HYPERTENSION AND BLOOD PRESSURE CONTROL

U.S. Federal Government/National Institutes of Health
www.nhlbi.nih.gov

DIABETES INFORMATION

www.diabetes.org/am2000

CARDIOLOGY AND HEART HEALTH

American Heart Association
www.theheart.org (General information.)
www.onelife.americanheart.org (Personalized program.)

HEART INFORMATION NETWORK

www.heartinfo.org

Cholstech
www.WellCheck.com (General and personalized information.)

HEALTH PROVIDERS RATING SERVICE

Health Grades
www.healthgrades.com (Ratings for hospitals and physicians.)

HEALTH INFORMATION: EVERYTHING BUT THE KITCHEN SINK

U.S. Federal Government/Health and Human Services
www.healthfinder.com (You could spend a week here!)

HEALTHY LIFESTYLE FOR SENIORS

www.silverfoxes.com (I contribute a heart-health column.)

A WORD OF CAUTION

I would place virtually zero trust in what might be picked up in an Internet chat room. You have no idea who those people are. Stick with established, proven sources of information.

RATING YOUR DOCTORS AND SURGEONS

When you place your health and your life in the hands of doctors, it's obviously wise to check on their past performances. This is the place to get that done: www.healthgrades.com.

15
To Tomorrow and Tomorrow and Tomorrow

It's funny how you remember some things just as clearly as though they'd happened just the other day. It was in 1986, when I was putting the finishing touches on my book and writing a little concluding chapter in which I tried to summarize my strong emotions about life, love, and health. I remember sitting at the same desk I'm at right now, with all sorts of memories and feelings crashing around in my head.

And here I am, more than a decade later, doing the last chapter for this new book. It deserves the same title I gave it last time, since this is one area of thought that hasn't changed much if at all over the intervening years.

Back in 1986 I was filled with hope that the program I had developed would indeed keep me around long enough to raise my children, Ross and Jenny. Today I still have that hope, only now I hope to be a part of my future grandchildren's lives. And that hope shares a place in my heart with the most profound gratitude that I have survived my fight with heart disease and have been able to help others do the same over the years.

My love for my children, and for my wife, Dawn, has grown through the years. Ross and Jenny are no longer little kids, but I know they still need me and want me to be around for many years to come.

I had a bittersweet experience in 1999 when I celebrated my fifty-seventh birthday. It was at that age that my own father passed away, after a massive heart attack. It was an eerie feeling to realize that I had reached his age. And I remember very well the day of his death. I was 26 at the time, and Dad and I were very close. I still miss him very much.

And that love for my father gets funneled into resolve to keep doing everything I can to preserve my own life so I can be around for my children. Wow, if only Dad could have lived to meet Ross and Jenny!

And, hey, my fight against heart disease isn't exactly the toughest thing a man has had to do. It's not battling in some foreign land with bullets flying. No, my fight—and yours—is a whole lot easier. All I have to do is get to the gym in the morning, stick with a low-fat diet rich in soluble fiber, take a few supplements with breakfast, lunch, and dinner, and see my doctors now and then for appropriate testing. Piece of cake, really.

In 1986 I wrote that, sure, I missed those greasy cheeseburgers and fries, barbecued pork ribs, and gooey pieces of chocolate cake. But giving up those things was never a problem when I thought of missing one of Ross's baseball games or Jenny's birthday parties. It all seemed so simple to me, that kind of choice. And it still does.

Of course, today my diet's a whole lot easier to follow. The phytosterols allow me to enjoy eggs on a weekend morning. I can prepare barbecued ribs with the special Piedmontese beef. Restrictions on polyunsaturated and monounsaturated fats like olive oil and nuts and avocados have been lifted.

But I still miss some of the foods that remain on the no-no list. So what? What double-cheese pizza could be a fair trade for not being around to witness the coming chapters in my family's life?

I'm a very lucky person. And so are you. Which brings me to the question I've never been able to figure out during the years I've been trying to help others fight heart disease: How can anyone, figuratively speaking, stand on the tracks while a train's bearing down on him, whistles blowing to get out of the way?

I want to grab such individuals by the proverbial lapels and shake them into reality. "Don't you realize that heart disease is serious, and that death is forever?" I want to scream.

Those who have suffered a heart attack know how willing they are to make any deals, at that moment of realization that death may be imminent, to stay alive. Those who do survive diligently watch their diets, take their prescribed medications, do some exercise—for a while. Then the memories and the fears fade, and it's back to the bad old ways.

One man I spoke with had had a major heart attack he was lucky to survive and had diabetes that, his doctors told him, could likely result in amputation of his feet if he didn't lose weight and start exercising. This was a man who, like me, loved his wife and children and had a very nice life. He said he wished he had my motivation. *What?* How much motivation does any human being need? Weren't his attractive wife and wonderful kids reason enough to make the needed lifestyle changes? Apparently not. The man was, quite literally, trading them in for a sack of doughnuts.

Of course, life isn't always a bed of roses. We all have our disappointments and our tragic moments. There are ups, there are downs. But on balance, this is the only game in town and we all have to make the most of it.

Have you really taken some time to count your own blessings? Have you made a mental list of the persons, places, and things you really like and love? By the mere fact that you're reading this book, I know you care about your health. So the ball is now in your court. You've got the information you need. You know the steps to take. As the Nike advertisement says, "Just do it!"

About a year after the book came out in 1987, I got a phone call from a man in Ohio. I have no idea how he got the number. He told me his wife had given him the book and he had read it on a business trip the week before. On the return flight home, he came to this chapter, and he started to think about his own wife and two little children. He said tears came to his eyes, and he made the decision to follow my example. Wow, that phone call meant a lot to me, and tears came to my own eyes as I spoke with him.

What's your reason for tomorrow? And tomorrow? And tomorrow?

Make your commitment today to a heart-healthy lifestyle. And keep up to date on all that's happening through my newsletter. I'll be there for you. Welcome to my special, very extended family!

16
Recipes That Lower Cholesterol

For too many years we've heard about "bad" foods that raise our cholesterol counts. But as I've pointed out throughout this book, there are foods that actually lower the amount of fats in our bloodstreams. That's particularly true for those rich in soluble fiber.

So how can we get more soluble fibers into our diets other than by eating bowl after bowl of oat bran and oatmeal? First, we go beyond oats to beans of all kinds, prunes, and other foods. And we can think of delicious ways to get that oat bran into lots of delicious treats.

Back in the 1980s, I tried every way imaginable to bake and cook with as little oil as possible. I even used corn syrup in baking my oat bran muffins since the syrup looked and felt like oil! Okay, those muffins weren't too bad, and they sure did a lot of good. Today, however, we know that corn, canola, and olive oils can be a part of a heart-healthy diet without raising cholesterol levels one bit. In fact, it's better to have more of the monounsaturated fats in our diets in order to keep our HDLs up and our triglycerides down.

Some of the recipes in this chapter are completely new, while others are updated for the new millennium. All of them are good, and good for you, and I hope you enjoy them as much as we do in our family.

So let's start where it all began for me—with oat bran. I called them "miracle muffins" when I described my daily breakfast blast of oat bran. Today they're just as effective and they taste a lot better.

OAT BRAN FOR LIFE

■ ■ ■ ■ ■ ■ ■ ■ ■ ■ ■ *Millennium Miracle Muffins*

2¼ cups oat bran cereal
¼ cup chopped nuts of your
   choice (a bit more if you
   like)
¼ cup raisins or other dried
   fruit
1 tbsp baking powder
¼ cup brown sugar, honey, or
   molasses
1¼ cups skim milk
4 oz egg substitute or
   2 beaten eggs*
3 tbsp canola oil

* If using whole eggs, be sure to swallow a phytosterol tablet before eating a muffin, or spread the muffin with a phytosterol-laced margarine.

Preheat the oven to 425°F. In a large bowl combine the oat bran, nuts, raisins, and baking powder. Stir in the sugar or other sweetening. Mix the milk, eggs, and oil together and blend in with the oat bran mixture. Line muffin pan with paper baking cups, and fill with batter. Bake 15 to 17 minutes. Test for doneness with a toothpick; it should come out moist but not wet. *Makes 12 muffins.*

■ ■ ■ ■ ■ ■ ■ ■ ■ ■ ■ *Apple Cinnamon Muffins*

1 cup skim milk
¼ cup frozen apple juice
   concentrate
4 oz egg substitute or
   2 beaten eggs
3 tbsp canola oil
2¼ cups oat bran cereal
¼ cup brown sugar
1¼ tsp cinnamon
1 tbsp baking powder
⅓ cup chopped walnuts
¼ cup raisins
1 medium apple, cored and
   chopped

Preheat the oven to 425°F. In a large bowl combine the milk, apple juice concentrate, eggs, and oil. Add the dry ingredients and mix. Blend in the chopped apple. Line muffin pan with paper baking cups, and fill with batter. Bake 15 to 17 minutes. *Makes 12 muffins.*

■ ■ ■ ■ ■ ■ ■ ■ ■ ■ ■ *Banana Nut Muffins*

2¼ cups oat bran cereal
1 tbsp baking powder
¼ cup brown sugar
½ cup chopped walnuts or
pecans
1¼ cups skim milk
2 ripe bananas, mashed
4 oz egg substitute or
2 beaten eggs
3 tbsp canola oil

Preheat the oven to 425°F. Mix
dry ingredients in a large bowl.
Mix milk, bananas, eggs, and oil
in a separate bowl, then add to dry
ingredients and blend. Line muffin
pan with paper baking cups, and
fill with batter. Bake for 15 to
17 minutes. *Makes 12 muffins.*

■ ■ ■ ■ ■ ■ ■ ■ ■ ■ ■ *Oatmeal Cookies*

1 cup canola oil
1 tsp vanilla extract
4 oz egg substitute or
2 beaten eggs
1½ cups brown sugar
2 cups rolled oats
2 cups oat bran
1 cup all-purpose flour
½ tsp baking soda
1 cup raisins (or mixture of
raisins and nuts)

*Here's the return of an old-
fashioned family treat. Enjoy one
or two in the evening with a nice
glass of cold milk.*

Preheat oven to 350°F. Mix moist
ingredients and sugar in a large
bowl, and gradually blend in dry
ingredients. Drop spoonfuls of
mixture onto a cookie pan lightly
sprayed with Baker's Joy. Bake
15 to 17 minutes or until edges are
browned. *Makes about 24 large,
36 medium, or up to 60 small
cookies.*

■ ■ ■ ■ ■ ■ ■ ■ ■ ■ ■ *Chocolate Chip 'n' Nuts
Cookies*

½ cup canola oil
1 tsp vanilla extract
2 oz egg substitutes or
2 beaten eggs
⅓ cup granulated sugar
⅓ cup brown sugar
2 cups oat bran
¾ cup self-rising flour

Preheat oven to 350°F. Mix canola
oil, vanilla extract, eggs, and
sugars until creamy. Add dry
ingredients in the order listed.
Drop with a spoon onto a cookie
sheet sprayed lightly with Baker's
Joy. Bake about 15 minutes or
until edges are slightly browned.

2 tsp baking powder
¼ cup chocolate chip morsels
½ cup chopped nuts

The larger the cookie, the longer the baking time. *Makes up to 36 cookies.*

■ ■ ■ ■ ■ ■ ■ ■ ■ ■ ■ *Peanut Butter Cookies*

½ cup peanut oil
1 cup chunk-style peanut butter
4 oz egg substitute or 2 beaten eggs
½ cup brown sugar
½ cup granulated sugar
2 cups oat bran
1 cup self-rising flour
1 tsp baking powder

This is real baking fun! It's my favorite cookie, but I avoided peanut butter cookies for years. Then we learned that nuts are actually good for us. This recipe also provides soluble fiber.

In a large bowl, blend the oil with the peanut butter and eggs until creamy. Gradually add the sugars, then mix in the dry ingredients. This is a heavy batter, and you may wish to use your hands to mix it. Chill the batter in the refrigerator for at least 2 hours or overnight. (You can keep the batter in the refrigerator for a week or more.)

Preheat oven to 350°F. Remove the batter one handful at a time from refrigerator to keep the rest cool, and form into walnut-size balls. Place on a cookie sheet and press down with a flour-dusted fork to form the cookie and give it the traditional crisscross pattern. Bake for 12 to 15 minutes or until browned at the edges. *Makes 24 cookies.*

■ ■ ■ ■ ■ ■ ■ ■ ■ ■ ■ *Fudge Brownies*

3 *tbsp cocoa*
1 *tbsp instant coffee*
1 *tbsp canola oil*
2 *ripe bananas, mashed*
2 *cups granulated sugar*
6 *oz egg substitute or*
   3 beaten eggs
1 *tsp rum extract*
1 *cup oat bran*
1/3 *cup chopped walnuts*

Preheat oven to 350°F. Mix cocoa, coffee, oil, and bananas in large bowl until well blended. Add sugar, eggs, and rum extract. Stir in oat bran and nuts. Pour into a 9-inch pan sprayed lightly with Baker's Joy. Bake 45 minutes. Cook and cut into 9 brownies.

These brownies are actually better for you than the fat-free commercially baked versions. The oil and nuts make them a lot more satisfying, and you won't be as tempted to overeat. Enjoy with a tall glass of cold milk.

MORE SOLUBLE FIBER

These are a few recipes to get you started baking with oat bran, but don't stop there. It's easy to simply add some oat bran to all your own favorite recipes by substituting for a portion of the flour. Next, I've got two terrific dessert ideas for you that provide some "hidden" soluble fibers.

■ ■ ■ ■ ■ ■ ■ ■ ■ ■ ■ *Chilled Prunes and Melon Balls*

1/2 *cup pitted prunes*
2 *cups Marsala or*
   sweet vermouth
1 *large ripe cantaloupe,*
   halved and seeded

This refreshing dessert comes from Italy. It's another good example of healthy Mediterranean food.

Cover the prunes with Marsala in a mixing bowl and marinate at room temperature for at least 1 hour. Use a melon baller to carve out the cantaloupe. Mix melon with prunes, and chill at least 1 hour before serving. Serve with a sprig of mint if you'd like to get fancy.

If you don't consume alcohol, you can replace the liquor with cherry or pomegranate juice.

■ ■ ■ ■ ■ ■ ■ ■ ■ ■ ■ *Baked Apples*

½ *cup raisins*
2 *tbsp dark rum (Meyers)*
1 *tbsp vanilla extract*
½ *cup very hot water*
2 *tbsp chopped walnuts*
1 *tbsp grated lemon rind*
1 *pinch cinnamon*
3 *tbsp honey*
1 *pinch ground cloves*
4 *large Granny Smith apples, cored but not peeled*

Preheat oven to 325°F. Mix raisins, rum, and vanilla extract with the hot water in a small bowl and let stand 30 minutes. Drain and reserve excess fluid. Mix walnuts, raisins, lemon rind, cinnamon, honey, and cloves and stuff into the apple cavities. Pierce apple skins to prevent bubbling. Drizzle apples with honey and place them in an oven-proof baking dish with fluid from the raisins. Cover with foil and bake 45 minutes to 1 hour, until apples are tender. Serve in shallow dishes with juices poured over. (Optional: Spritz apples with nonfat or reduced-fat whipped cream.)

DINNER SALADS

Typical salads are often "junk food" with nothing more than nutrient-free iceberg lettuce and high-calorie dressings. Create wonderful salads by using a wide variety of greens and chopped vegetables and fruits. Try some chopped figs, dates, and raisins to contribute a bit of contrasting sweetness.

Add soluble fiber to almost any salad by adding various kinds of beans. Garbanzos (chick peas) are always good. White Italian beans (cannellini) are terrific in antipasto salads. Red kidney beans are a nice change of pace. Here's a recipe for a great three-bean salad.

■ ■ ■ ■ ■ ■ ■ ■ ■ ■ ■ *Ultimate Three-Bean Salad*

$\frac{1}{3}$ cup granulated sugar
$\frac{1}{3}$ cup canola oil
$\frac{3}{4}$ cup red wine vinegar
1 tsp salt
1 16-oz can cut
  green beans, drained
1 16-oz can garbanzo
  beans, drained
1 16-oz can red kidney
  beans, drained
$\frac{1}{2}$ cup chopped red onions

Combine sugar, oil, vinegar, and salt in a large bowl. Add beans and onions and toss to coat thoroughly. Refrigerate in a large, covered container with a good seal, at least overnight. Turn the container every couple of hours or so, when you think about it, to develop the full flavor. This recipe is ridiculously simple, yet I'll bet it's the best you've ever had.

SOUP

What happens when you take these kinds of ingredients and cook them in liquid? Why, soup, of course. Studies have demonstrated that soups are actually far more satisfying than salads, even when the identical ingredients are used. I prefer starting meals with soups rather than salads, so I might be a bit prejudiced. Here are a few of my own favorites.

■ ■ ■ ■ ■ ■ ■ ■ ■ ■ ■ *Pasta e Fagioli Zuppa*

1 cup chopped onion
1 cup chopped carrots
1 cup chopped celery
$\frac{1}{2}$ cup chopped red bell
  pepper
2 tbsp olive oil
2 cups water
2 cups cooked elbow
  macaroni
$\frac{1}{4}$ cup chopped parsley
  (Italian if available)
$\frac{1}{3}$ tsp thyme
$\frac{1}{4}$ tsp salt
$\frac{1}{2}$ tsp pepper
  (freshly ground if possible)
1 16-oz can cannellini
  (Italian white beans)

That's Italian for pasta and bean soup. Italians I've known tend to call it "pasta fazzool." You'll call it delicious as a starter to any meal, Italian or not.

Sauté onion, carrots, celery, and bell pepper in olive oil until onion is transparent. Add 1 cup water and cook covered for about 15 minutes. Add remaining ingredients except for the cheese and cook another 10 minutes. Serve with grated parmesan cheese. (For a real flavor blast, try grating some fresh, imported parmesan. You'll need just a

1 14.5-oz can low-sodium
chicken broth
½ cup chopped, seeded
tomatoes
grated parmesan cheese

tablespoonful or so, so the
saturated fat is minimal.)

■ ■ ■ ■ ■ ■ ■ ■ ■ ■ ■ *Minestrone Soup*

1 medium onion, finely
chopped
2 carrots, chopped
2 celery stalks, chopped
2 tbsp olive oil
2 quarts low-sodium
chicken broth
1 medium potato, peeled
and diced
2 large ripe tomatoes,
seeded and diced
1 tbsp tomato paste
1 15-oz can white beans,
drained
½ head of cabbage, chopped
1 tsp Italian seasoning
2 bay leaves
½ 10-oz package frozen
spinach, or one bunch
fresh spinach, chopped
1 tbsp salt
½ tsp ground black pepper
(freshly ground is
preferred)
½ cup frozen green peas
7 oz elbow macaroni
(or other shaped pasta)

Sauté onion, carrots, and celery in
olive oil until onion is transparent.
Add broth, potato, and sautéed
vegetables to a large saucepan or
pot, along with all other
ingredients except peas and pasta.
Bring to a boil, reduce heat, and
simmer for about 1 hour. Add peas
and pasta, bring back to boil, and
simmer another 10 minutes.

Instead of the usual grated
parmesan cheese, try some
romano. Freshly grated is always
better.

Minestrone varies, region by
region, throughout Italy. This
recipe combines tastes from
Tuscany and Milan.

■ ■ ■ ■ ■ ■ ■ ■ ■ ■ ■ *Pea Soup*

1 medium onion, chopped
  fine
1 celery stalk, chopped fine
1 carrot, chopped
2 tbsp olive oil
1½ cups dried split peas,
  rinsed
4 cloves garlic, peeled and
  crushed
1½ quarts low-sodium
  chicken broth
¼ tsp ground sage
½ tsp thyme
½ tsp dried basil
12 caraway or anise seeds,
  crushed (your taste
  preference)
1 tsp salt
1 tsp freshly ground
  black pepper
1 cup frozen peas (thawed)
½ cup lean ham, cubed

This is the absolute winner for soluble fiber content. "Pease porridge hot, pease porridge cold, pease porridge in the pot, nine days old." So the children's poem goes. I don't know about cold pea soup, but I do know it gets better over time in the refrigerator. Here's a version that comes from France.

Sauté onion, celery, and carrots in olive oil in a large pot or dutch oven until onion is transparent. Add split peas, crushed garlic, chicken broth, herbs and seeds, salt, and pepper. Bring to boil, reduce heat, and simmer covered for about 1 hour. Add previously frozen peas. In batches, purée soup in a blender or, preferably, a food processor. Return to pot, stir in ham cubes, heat through, and serve.

■ ■ ■ ■ ■ ■ ■ ■ ■ ■ ■ *Soups Without Recipes*

I don't know about you, but I really prefer cooking without recipes whenever possible. It's more fun, lots faster than having to keep looking at the recipe, and I get to use up a lot of stuff in the refrigerator. So, instead of a recipe, here's a list of steps you can use to make your own soups. Each one will be slightly different, but they will all be delicious.

1. Sauté chopped onion, carrots, celery, bell peppers in olive oil in

a large pot. Want some zucchini instead of the celery? Go for it. Mix and match whatever you like.

2. Add about 1 quart of low-sodium chicken, beef, or vegetable broth.

3. Add some chunks of vegetables you like. Try some sweet potatoes for a different flavor and a wonderful dollop of beta-carotene and other antioxidants. Chop up some spinach or other greens. Maybe a turnip, parsnip, or rutabaga. Toss in ¼ tsp of this herb or that. Experiment.

4. Bring it all to a boil, reduce heat, and simmer an hour or so.

5. Add a can of drained beans of your choice: red or white kidney beans, great northern beans, or maybe lentils. Heat through for another 10 minutes.

6. Serve as is, or purée the soup first. Again, your choice.

7. Add a splash or two of Land o' Lakes fat-free half-and-half for marvelous creaminess.

BEANS, BEANS . . .

■ ■ ■ ■ ■ ■ ■ ■ ■ ■ ■ *Bob's Best Chili*

For years, my family and friends have marveled over my chili. And when I'm asked for the recipe, I get embarrassed because it's so simple. People usually expect more, some secret ingredient. But no, there's nothing to it. An easy, nutritious meal all by itself.

1. Start by browning a pound of extra-lean ground beef in a fairly large skillet. If it's ultralean, with virtually no fat of its own (the way I like it), brown the beef in 1 tbsp of heated canola oil. Keep poking at it with a wooden spoon so no big lumps form.
2. Whirl a large can of peeled tomatoes (I like Hunt's tomatoes) in a blender just long enough to form a slurry, with no big tomato pieces.
3. Add tomatoes to the beef, along with 2 (not 1, 2) cans of S&W Zesty Chili Beans, and a packet of Lawry's chili mix. (DO NOT substitute other brands—believe me, this makes the difference.)
4. Stir it all together, bring to a bubble, cover and simmer for 5 to 10 minutes.
5. Cook one 7-oz box of Creamette elbow macaroni and drain.
6. Serve chili over macaroni. Put out bowls of low-fat cheddar cheese shreds, nonfat sour cream, chopped onions, and oyster

crackers to choose from. (It's best with all the above.)

7. Enjoy both the chili and the compliments.

■ ■ ■ ■ ■ ■ ■ ■ ■ ■ ■ *Hummus (Garbanzo Bean Dip)*

½ *cup sesame tahini*
¼ *cup lemon juice*
5 *cloves garlic, minced (more if you prefer)*
5 *drops Tabasco*
¼ *cup water*
½ *tsp cumin*
2 *15-oz cans garbanzo beans (chick peas), drained*

After all these years, this remains one of my favorite recipes. Hummus makes a great appetizer or a quick snack. Enjoy with toasted wedges of pita bread. I've increased the sesame tahini a bit, and suggest you "float" a bit of extra-virgin olive oil on top when you serve it.

There's nothing to it. Simply combine all ingredients and blend in a food processor until smooth. Keep chilled in the refrigerator for up to two weeks for handy snacks that pack a whale of a lot of soluble fiber.

WHOOPS, WHERE'S THE NUTRITION INFORMATION?

No, I didn't forget to do a listing of calories and fat grams. We don't have to count those fat grams anymore, since only the saturated fats and trans fats raise cholesterol levels, and these recipes don't have offending ingredients. As to calories, by cutting down on fats and sugars, especially in fast foods and processed foods and fatty desserts, you won't have to worry about them either.

17
Cooking with the Kowalskis

I'm a little embarrassed when I look at the subtitle of the original book, which promises "no deprivation." Well, that's a bit of a stretch. All of us who wanted to follow a heart-healthy lifestyle certainly had to give up a lot of different foods back in those days. It sure is a lot easier today.

Then: Limit all fats; count those fat grams every day. Now: Limit only the saturated and trans fats; don't bother with counting. Then: Eliminate all whole eggs; use only whites and substitutes. Now: Block the absorption of dietary cholesterol by simply swallowing a phytosterol tablet or two. Then: Cut way back on red meat; use turkey instead. Now: Enjoy every cut of beef thanks to "designer" cattle.

If you were to come to dinner at our home, you'd be hard put to see many if any differences from the way most Americans eat. All of us in our family love food. It's a major part of our lives, both at home and in restaurants or on vacations. Our midwestern roots definitely show in dishes such as meatloaf, mashed potatoes, and gravy. What could define barbecue better than ribs with creamy potato salad? And, like most Americans, we've been influenced by regional food tastes: blackened fish from New Orleans, Mexican dishes from the Southwest, and Boston clam chowder made with cream, not skim milk. Yes, cream. Even that ingredient is available to you today. Definitely, positively, no deprivation!

Of course, this isn't a cookbook. It'd take at least one book, maybe more, to share my entire recipe file with you. But I'd like you to try some of our very favorites. And by seeing the way we cook and the ingredients we use, you'll be able to whip up your own favorites with the saturated fats pared way down.

A BIT OF PLANNING

A USDA survey done a few years ago revealed that the biggest stumbling block to more healthful eating patterns was lack of planning. Folks tend to come home from work hungry, look in the refrigerator, and wind up ordering a pizza. Or they try to throw something together at the last minute.

What I'd like to suggest will probably be the most foreign concept I've proposed in this book. Take a few moments to write down a plan for the week's meals. Then make a shopping list to provide all the ingredients you'll need.

Your first objection, I'm sure, will be the unpredictability of your family and yourself. Who knows who's going to be available for dinner this night or that? First, maybe it would be a good idea to schedule some time together for the family. Second, many menu ideas are pretty flexible, such that everyone need not sit down to the table at the same time. If you prepare my shepherd's pie, for example, you'll have a one-dish casserole you and others can dig into anytime during the evening.

Your second objection might be that you just don't have time to cook a meal every evening. Neither do I. Here's my suggestion. When you do have the time to prepare, let's say, a meatloaf, make three of them. Bake one for that evening, and put the other two away in the freezer, uncooked, for those particularly hectic days. After several days of doing this, you'll soon have a well-stocked freezer with meals of all sorts ready to simply thaw in the microwave and pop in the oven.

The next three times you go shopping, plan for an extra 20 minutes in the supermarket. That will give you the time to leisurely go down each aisle and take a few moments to compare one brand of this or that by reading the nutrition facts and ingredients labels. One study has shown that after three shopping trips, most people begin to repeat their purchases. By that time, then, you won't have to take the time to make your selections; you'll know exactly which ones are best.

But once in a while, perhaps once a month, view your shopping trip more as an adventure of discovery than a chore. Spend a little time in the produce section. Talk with the manager there about how to prepare a vegetable you may not have cooked before. Look at new items that have been added to the shelves. Finding just one such item can open the doors to a number of cooking possibilities. I remember when I first found the Land o' Lakes fat-free half-and-half. Suddenly my mashed potatoes went from pretty good to sinfully delicious, I was able to re-create a few old-fashioned creamy drinks, and on and on. (Of course, I also report on all such new food products in *The Diet-Heart Newsletter*.)

Try to keep a variety of foods in the refrigerator and freezer for spur-of-the-moment needs. Certainly you'll want to have some cold cuts for sandwiches and ingredients to put together an interesting salad.

SCRUMPTIOUS SOUPS AND SIDE DISHES

In the next few pages I think I'll convince you that the idea of boosting your daily vegetable intake sounds mighty delicious. These dishes make meals memorable.

■ ■ ■ ■ ■ ■ ■ ■ ■ ■ ■ *Jenny's Butternut Squash Soup*

2 *lbs butternut squash*
2 *cups chopped onion*
2 *tbsp olive oil*
4 *cups low-sodium chicken broth*
1 *tsp salt*
¾ *tsp curry powder*
¼ *tsp each ground nutmeg, white pepper, ground ginger*
2 *bay leaves*
½ *cup Land o' Lakes fat-free half-and-half*

My daughter Jenny enjoys cooking when she's home from college, and I always ask her to make this incredibly delicious soup for me when she comes for a visit. It's a bit complicated, but the result is worth the effort. You'll thank Jenny for inventing it.

Preheat oven to 350°F. Cut squash in half and scoop out the seeds. Place in casserole dish cut side down in about 1 inch of water. Bake for 40 to 45 minutes. Allow to cool, then remove skin and cut into chunks. (Prepare other ingredients while the squash is baking.)

Sauté onion in olive oil until transparent, about 3 to 4 minutes, over medium heat. Stir in the chunks of squash, chicken broth, and seasonings. Bring to boil in a suitably sized pot, reduce heat, and simmer 15 minutes.

Remove bay leaves and blend the soup in a food processor in batches. Return to pot, heat through, and add half-and-half.

You'll have a creamy soup that you and your friends would swear is loaded with fat. Serve with sprigs of basil, if you wish, for a festive touch. *Makes 8 servings.*

■ ■ ■ ■ ■ ■ ■ ■ ■ ■ ■ ■ **Generic Cream Soups**

Most of the time, I cook without recipes. To me, it's quicker and a lot more fun. So here's a generic approach to making a wide variety of cream soups. Make big batches so you'll have enough for dinner one night and lunch the next day.

1. Start with 4 cups of peeled, chunked potatoes (usually white but occasionally sweet) and cook until mushy in a quart of broth (usually chicken, but sometimes beef or vegetable).
2. When the potatoes start getting soft and split easily with a fork, add any of a variety of vegetables, including broccoli, cauliflower, asparagus (peeled to remove those little leaves), carrots, leeks, or beets. I usually use an equal amount of potatoes and vegetables, but you may prefer to go heavier on the veggies, or the other way around.
3. Continue cooking until vegetables are mushy. Season with herbs such as thyme, curry powder, dill, and allspice. Dill, for example, goes beautifully with

carrot soup. Curry and cauliflower were meant for each other. Thyme is great for broccoli and asparagus. Use about $\frac{1}{2}$ tsp. Season with salt and freshly ground pepper to taste.

4. Serve as is or blend in a food processor. If as is, add 3 tbsp of margarine (tub or squeeze). If blended, stir in $\frac{1}{2}$ cup of fat-free Land o' Lakes half-and-half.

5. If you happen to have some ham or low-fat sausage left over, this is a good time to use that meat. Stir it in and you'll have a meal in a bowl.

■ ■ ■ ■ ■ ■ ■ ■ ■ ■ ■ *Escarole Soup*

3 *quarts water*
1 *tbsp plus 1 tsp salt*
2 *tbsp lemon juice*
1 *large head of escarole (about 1¼ pounds), cleaned and chopped coarsely*
4 *cups chicken broth*
2 *cloves garlic, minced*
¼ *tsp freshly ground black pepper (more if you prefer)*
2 *tbsp grated parmesan cheese*

Italians are about the only nationality familiar with soups as vehicles for leafy green vegetables. This recipe calls specifically for escarole, but you could just as easily substitute spinach or other greens. Making this soup is so easy, I'm sure you'll do it again and again.

Bring water to a boil with 1 tbsp salt and lemon juice. Add escarole and bring to a boil. Reduce heat and simmer for 3 minutes. Drain and discard water. Add broth, garlic, 1 tsp salt, and pepper. Bring to a boil, reduce heat, and simmer 10 minutes. Serve with grated parmesan cheese.

■ ■ ■ ■ ■ ■ ■ ■ ■ ■ ■   ## California Sunshine Soup

1   quart Clamato juice
½   cup chopped cucumber
¼   pound cooked tiny cocktail shrimp
1   8-oz package fat-free or lite cream cheese cut into ½-inch cubes
1   medium avocado cut into ½-inch cubes
⅓   cup sweet onion, chopped fine
2   tbsp olive oil
2   tbsp red wine vinegar
1   tbsp sugar
1   large garlic clove, minced (more if you prefer)
⅓   tsp Tabasco sauce

Here's another "blast from the past"—from the original book but brought up to speed for the millennium. It's great on a hot summer day, perhaps with a sandwich, when it's too hot to cook.

Mix all ingredients in a large, sealed container and refrigerate at least overnight to bring out all the flavors. That's critical. Do not serve immediately.

■ ■ ■ ■ ■ ■ ■ ■ ■ ■ ■   ## Colonel Kowalski's Coleslaw

½   cup granulated sugar
½   tsp salt
¼   tsp ground white pepper
½   cup light mayonnaise (1 gram of fat per tablespoon)*
½   cup low-fat (1%) buttermilk
1½   tsp white vinegar
2½   tbsp lemon juice
8   cups cabbage, chopped fine
½   cup carrots, chopped fine

I call it that because it's similar to that served at Kentucky Fried Chicken, but with a lot less fat. Another mighty tasty way to get some veggies into your day. Enjoy it with a sandwich when there's no time to cook.

Combine all ingredients except cabbage and carrots, then mix in the veggies. Important: Chop very fine. Refrigerate in a sealed plastic container.

*Don't try to save fat by getting the fat-free mayos on the market; they just don't taste good. I like the Hellman's/Best Foods low-fat mayonnaise with just 1 gram of fat per tablespoon. And none of that fat is the saturated or trans artery-clogging type.

■ ■ ■ ■ ■ ■ ■ ■ ■ ■ ■ *Hollywood Cobb Salad*

2 cups mixed greens (iceberg, romaine, bibb), chopped fine
½ cup each mushrooms, broccoli, carrots, chopped fine
¼ cup each sweet onions, beets, bell pepper

The famous Brown Derby restaurant closed its doors just after I got here in 1980. But it left a wonderful legacy in the cob salad, now served in restaurants widely. It's best when veggies are chopped fine and they all blend together.

This recipe yields enough for two people. Multiply ingredients for more people. How about making it for your Academy Awards party? Or perhaps to bring along for a picnic?

Combine all ingredients and mix well in a large ziplock bag. Keep chilled until ready to serve with the dressing of your choice.

■ ■ ■ ■ ■ ■ ■ ■ ■ ■ ■ *Sweet Potato Salad*

2 large sweet potatoes or yams
water to cover
1 cup celery, diced
1 cup apples, diced
⅓ cup walnuts, chopped
¼ cup low-fat mayonnaise (Hellman's/Best Foods)
2 tbsp sugar
2 tbsp lemon juice
½ tsp salt

Sweet potatoes are packed with both vitamin C and beta-carotene. Here's a great way to enjoy them.

Peel and cut sweet potatoes into chunks. Bring to a boil in a pot with enough water to cover them, and cook until tender but not mushy. While potatoes cook, prepare other ingredients and mix in a plastic container. Add potatoes when they've cooled after cooking and draining.

■ ■ ■ ■ ■ ■ ■ ■ ■ ■ ■ *Carrot Salad*

 1 lb carrots, shredded
½ cup raisins
½ cup celery, diced
 1 tsp lemon juice
 1 tsp granulated sugar
½ cup low-fat mayonnaise
     (Hellman's/Best Foods)

Ah, another great source of beta-carotene, along with all the other carotenoids that do our hearts good. It happens to be one of my favorites, so I hope you'll enjoy it as well.

Nothing to it. Just mix all ingredients. You can shred the carrots with your food processor or by hand with a grater.

■ ■ ■ ■ ■ ■ ■ ■ ■ ■ ■ *Classic Potato Salad*

 5 lbs red potatoes
salted water
 1 each medium red and
     green bell peppers, diced
 5 stalks celery, diced
12 large green olives with
     pimentos, sliced
 6 hard-cooked eggs (or
     12 whites only)
 1 tsp salt
½ cup low-fat mayonnaise
     (Hellman's/Best Foods)
½ tsp paprika

I'm no doubt biased toward this recipe, since it's the one I've enjoyed as a child. I think my mom made a great potato salad. For a long time, I used only the egg whites, but now I use yolks as well, thanks to the phytosterols that block the absorption of cholesterol. All the flavor's back!

Boil potatoes in salted water in their skins until tender to fork, about 15 minutes. While the potatoes cook, dice the peppers, celery, olives, and eggs. Drain and allow potatoes to cool, then peel off skins and cut into chunks. Mix all these ingredients in a large plastic container. Add the mayonnaise. (I use my hands to do the mixing.) Top off with the paprika.

■ ■ ■ ■ ■ ■ ■ ■ ■ ■ ■ *Dinner Salad*

Salad should be an opportunity to get two or three vegetable/fruit servings into the day's fare. Not just iceberg lettuce. I like to keep ingredients chopped and prepared in containers in the refrigerator so they're handy. Start with mixed greens, including romaine, bibb, red or green leaf lettuce, and spinach. Then add the goodies. Finish with dressing of your choice. Goodie list: beets, shredded carrots, julienned bell peppers, olives, broccoli florets, cauliflower, tomatoes, radishes, celery, green onion, avocado, orange segments, raisins, nuts.

■ ■ ■ ■ ■ ■ ■ ■ ■ ■ ■ *Sweet Potato Supreme*

1 *lb sweet potatoes or yams*
   (3 medium, 2 large)
salted water
½ *cup fat-free sour cream*
2 *oz egg substitute*
½ *tsp salt*
¼ *tsp mace*
¾ *cup miniature*
   marshmallows

The easiest way to enjoy sweet potatoes, and one we do a lot, is to simply microwave them. But now and then you may want something a little fancier. This dish is perfect along with ham or turkey. I make one or two extra to freeze; do so before baking. This was inspired by a classic Betty Crocker recipe.

Boil potatoes in salted water until very soft but not mushy. Drain. Preheat oven to 350°F. Combine potatoes or yams with all other ingredients except marshmallows, and blend until smooth with a hand mixer. Spray casserole dish with Pam or other vegetable oil cooking spray and ladle in the mixture. Top with marshmallows. Bake 30 minutes. Marshmallows should be browned.

■ ■ ■ ■ ■ ■ ■ ■ ■ ■ ■ *Roasted Vegetables*

Sweet potatoes might be one of the many vegetables you could roast as an alternative to dull and boring boiling or steaming. Peel and cut into chunks, then toss with a generous drizzle of olive oil, seasoned with salt, pepper, and a little nutmeg or cinnamon. Roast in a preheated 400°F oven for about 30 minutes or until nice and tender.

Other vegetables to consider for roasting include asparagus, broccoli, cauliflower, beets, and such roots as parsnips and turnips, as well as green beans. Or combine 2 or more. Again, toss with some olive oil along with salt and pepper and seasonings such as thyme. Roasting at 400°F takes 20 to 30 minutes, depending on the veggie.

■ ■ ■ ■ ■ ■ ■ ■ ■ ■ ■ *Sautéed Vegetables*

This method is even easier and takes less time than roasting. Start with 1 or 2 tbsp of olive oil. Then pick your veggie for the evening: asparagus, bell peppers (combine colors), fennel, onions, carrots sliced into sticks about the thickness of a pencil, or leeks. Try combinations. Peppers and sweet onions are delicious together. Simply sauté in olive oil until tender. Season with salt and pepper if you like.

■ ■ ■ ■ ■ ■ ■ ■ ■ ■ ■ *Microwaved Acorn Squash*

Everyone in my family looks forward to this easy-to-prepare side dish. Cut an acorn squash in half, and remove the seeds and strings. Pierce the flesh with a fork repeatedly. With your fingers, smear a little margarine (tub or squeeze) into the cavities. Sprinkle with brown sugar. Microwave on high for 10 minutes. Using a fork or spoon, break up flesh and mix in the margarine and brown sugar. Return to microwave for another 5 minutes. Count on 1 squash for 2 persons.

■ ■ ■ ■ ■ ■ ■ ■ ■ ■ ■ *Garlic Spinach*

1   *cup water*
2   *lbs fresh spinach, cleaned and stems removed*
2   *tsp extra-virgin olive oil*
2   *cloves garlic, minced*
1   *tsp lemon juice*
$\frac{1}{4}$ *tsp salt*
$\frac{1}{4}$ *tsp freshly ground pepper*

Bring water to boil in medium saucepan or other pot. Drop in cleaned spinach leaves and stir, swirling in the water for no more than 2 minutes to par-cook it. Heat olive oil in skillet and sauté garlic until tender, about 2 minutes. Add spinach to skillet and sauté another 2 to 3 minutes or until spinach is tender and softened. Drizzle lemon juice and dash with salt and pepper.

■ ■ ■ ■ ■ ■ ■ ■ ■ ■ ■ *Parslied Carrots*

4 *medium carrots, peeled*
    and sliced as you like them
½ *tbsp olive oil*
½ *tsp sugar*
2 *cloves garlic, minced*
2 *tbsp parsley, chopped,*
    stems removed
¼ *tsp salt*
¼ *tsp pepper*

Blanch carrots in boiling water for 5 minutes. Drain and set aside carrots. Heat olive oil with sugar in a skillet. Sauté garlic for 2 minutes. Add carrots and sauté for 5 minutes. Stir in parsley, season with salt and pepper, remove from heat, and serve.

■ ■ ■ ■ ■ ■ ■ ■ ■ ■ ■ *Mashed Potatoes*

2 *lbs (two large) potatoes,*
    peeled and chunked
water (or low-sodium
    chicken broth)
2 *tbsp squeeze-bottle*
    *margarine**
⅓ *cup Land o' Lakes fat-free*
    half-and-half
salt and pepper to taste

*I use Fleischmann's Light squeeze-bottle margarine. It has 6 grams of fat per tablespoon, none of which is either saturated or trans. The oil is not hydrogenated.

Potatoes were a staple of my childhood diet. We had mashed spuds most nights of the week. But without butter and cream, or at least whole milk, they lost a lot of sparkle for many years. Now, with new ingredients, I'm in my glory again. In fact, I make very big batches and freeze portions for spur-of-the-moment use. Multiply this recipe as needed.

Bring potatoes to a boil in a pot with enough water to cover. Reduce heat slightly and cook until tender to a fork. Drain. Mash with hand mixer. Add margarine and continue to mash. Add half-and-half and salt and pepper, and finish mashing.

For variety and to double the fiber, leave skins on. Scrub under running water to clean. Then chunk and cook as usual.

MAIN DISHES, FROM MEATS TO FISHES

Happy days are here again! Even the American Heart Association now advocates eating fish, especially fatty fish, at least twice weekly. The shellfish once avoided because of supposedly high levels of cholesterol have been found to be not only virtually fat-free but also very low in cholesterol.

Modern ranchers have improved beef and pork. Lowest-fat cuts have the words "loin" or "round" in their names. Some cattle produce meat with no more fat than chicken in *all* cuts, making it possible to enjoy normally fatty cuts such as ribs and brisket. For sources of lean meat, see "Listening to Your Inner Carnivore" in Chapter 4.

Some pork producers have bred their hogs to be leaner than ever. Smithfield is a great brand to look for. Choose low-fat cuts including pork loin, tenderloin, and ham or Canadian bacon. When you see pork loin on sale, have the butcher trim and grind it for use in meatballs and meatloaf.

Unless you have ethical problems with veal, choose this red meat, which is naturally low in fat, extremely tender, and a wonderful taste contribution to your dishes. Think of all the Italian dishes alone: veal scallopini, parmesano, and picante. Start with a crisp salad or a minestrone soup. Match with a side dish of pasta and some vegetables, and enjoy with a nice bottle of chianti. *Mangia!* (That's Italian for Enjoy!)

■ ■ ■ ■ ■ ■ ■ ■ ■ ■ ■ *Bob's Special Meatloaf*

1 *lb extralean ground beef*
½ *lb lean ground pork*
1 *cup bread crumbs*
3½ *tbsp ketchup*
1 *beaten egg or 2 oz egg
   substitute*
1½ *tbsp Worcestershire sauce*
¼ *tsp each sage, ground
   pepper, marjoram,
   celery salt*
½ *tsp salt*
2 *garlic cloves, minced*
¼ *tsp dijon mustard*
½ *green pepper, chopped fine*
3 *slices onion, chopped fine*
6 *green olives, chopped*
½ *red pepper, sliced into
   strips*

Preheat oven to 350°F. Mix meat and moist ingredients in a large bowl. Separately mix dry ingredients and then add to meat mixture. Form the loaf. Decorate top with sliced red pepper. Bake in casserole dish for about 1 hour or until meat thermometer reads 160°F. Let stand for 5 minutes, slice, and serve.

Remember: they don't call it beefloaf, it's meatloaf. So mixing the pork with beef really makes a taste difference. Serve with mashed potatoes, of course, and plenty of gravy. For the latter, combine a packet each of brown and pork gravy mix with 2 cups of water in the casserole dish while the meatloaf is resting, along with the cooked juices. Bring to a boil on the stovetop, simmer for 5 minutes.

Spectacular Meat Loaf

3/4 cup each minced onion
and green onion
1/2 cup each minced celery
and carrot
1/4 cup each minced green
pepper and red pepper
2 tsp minced garlic cloves
2 tbsp olive oil
1 tsp salt (and freshly
ground pepper to taste)
1/2 tsp each ground cumin and
nutmeg
1/4 tsp cayenne pepper
1/2 cup ketchup
4 oz egg substitute or
2 beaten eggs
1/2 cup Land o' Lakes fat-free
half-and-half
1 pound each lean ground
beef and pork
3/4 cup oat bran

I first published this recipe in The
8-Week Cholesterol Cure. Here it is
again, with a few modifications to
bring it up to date. This takes some
time to prepare, but it's really
worth it. You can even serve it to
company with pride.

Preheat oven to 350°F. Sauté
vegetables until tender in olive oil.
Set aside to cool in a large mixing
bowl. Add herbs and seasonings.
Next add ketchup, eggs, and half-
and-half, followed by the blended
ground meats, and finally the oat
bran. Mix well and form into 1 or
2 loaves. Place in baking pan and
bake for 50 to 55 minutes.

Spectacular Meatloaf Sauce

8 medium-sized shallots,
minced
3 tbsp olive oil
1 tbsp ground thyme
3 bay leaves
1/2 tsp crushed black
peppercorns
2 cups each dry white wine,
chicken broth, and beef
broth

While the meatloaf is baking, it's
time to prepare the sauce.

Sauté shallots in olive oil along
with herbs and pepper until tender
Add wine and reduce to a glaze
over high heat. Add beef and
chicken broths and bring to a boil.
Reduce heat and cook until
reduced to 2 cups.

Serve with mashed potatoes
and a side dish of spinach.

■ ■ ■ ■ ■ ■ ■ ■ ■ ■ ■ *Swedish Meatballs*

1½ *slices white bread with*
crusts trimmed
½ *cup Land o' Lakes fat-free*
half-and-half
2 *oz egg substitute or*
1 beaten egg
½ *tsp vinegar*
¼ *tsp nutmeg*
½ *cup fresh dill, minced*
1 *tsp each salt and pepper*
½ *lb each lean ground beef,*
pork, and veal
1 *medium onion, minced*
2 *tbsp canola oil*
1 *cup nonfat sour cream*
¼ *cup dry sherry*
½ *cup beef broth*

Soak bread in half-and-half and work together with your fingers or a spoon until you have mush. Add egg, vinegar, nutmeg, half the minced dill, and salt and pepper. Next add blended meats and minced onion and blend well. (Using your hands is easiest.) Form into walnut-sized meatballs. (Perhaps you'll want to freeze half for another time.) Fry the meatballs in a skillet with heated canola oil.

While the meatballs are frying, mix the remaining dill with the sour cream in one container (I use a measuring cup) and the sherry and beef broth in another. Remove the fried meatballs and pour the sherry-broth mixture into the hot pan to deglaze it. With the ensuing sizzle, make a gravy as you scrape the bits off the bottom of the pan. Return the meatballs to that sauce and warm through. Finally, add the dill–sour cream mix and blend. (Make sure that the meatballs and sauce are only warm, not hot, so the sour cream doesn't crack.)

Serve with noodles and carrots.

■ ■ ■ ■ ■ ■ ■ ■ ■ ■ ■ *Pepper Stroganoff Steak*

1 lb low-fat beef cut into
   $\frac{1}{2}$-inch strips
1 tbsp canola oil
1 packet dried onion soup
   mix
$\frac{1}{4}$ cup water
2 bay leaves
1 can (10$\frac{3}{4}$-oz) low-fat
   cream of tomato soup
2 large bell peppers cut into
   strips
2 tbsp nonfat sour cream

This isn't pepper steak by ordinary definitions. It's more like a stroganoff with bell peppers. But my mom always called it a pepper steak. Unfortunately I had to give it up for a few years until nonfat sour cream and reduced-fat cream of tomato soup came on the market. The lowest-fat version will call for Belgian Blue or Piedmontese beef, but you can trim off the fat from a lean chunk of chuck steak from the supermarket. This is bound to become one of your family's favorites, as it is in ours.

In a heavy skillet that has a cover, brown meat in oil. Add dried onion soup mix and water, stir, cover, and simmer 1 hour or until tender. Add bay leaves, tomato soup, and a little more water if needed. Simmer 15 minutes. Add bell pepper strips and simmer a final 15 minutes. Remove from heat and allow to cool down a bit before adding the sour cream so it doesn't crack. Serve with noodles.

■ ■ ■ ■ ■ ■ ■ ■ ■ ■ ■ *Just Plain Steak*

*When you don't have time or incli-
nation to do anything fancy, it's
time for a steak. This is when you
want to have some Belgian Blue or
Piedmontese beef steaks in the
freezer. I keep a good supply of
ribeyes, New York strips, and
porterhouse steaks, which I serve
about once a week. I order them
nice and thick, so they can be
cooked rare on the inside and
charred on the outside.*

Start with a crisp salad. Then settle
into your steak with a vegetable
dish (we love asparagus simply
steamed and drizzled with extra-
virgin olive oil), a baked potato
(stick a couple into the oven at
400°F for an hour while you're
getting everything else ready),
perhaps a chunk of crusty bread,
and, by all means, a good glass of
red wine.

This meal is practically zero
effort, with a huge payoff in taste
and enjoyment. To thaw steaks
straight from the freezer, put them
in a basin of water while the
potatoes bake. Get everything
started when you walk in the door,
and by the time you've greeted the
family, gone through your mail,
and taken a shower, you'll be
ready to go.

■ ■ ■ ■ ■ ■ ■ ■ ■ ■ *Barbecued Ribs*

1 *lb beef ribs (typically*
   3 ribs) per person
water
4 *bay leaves*
1 *tbsp black peppercorns*
4 *garlic cloves, peeled and*
   crushed
2 *tbsp vinegar*
barbecue sauce of your choice

Thanks to that "designer" beef I can once again enjoy juicy barbecued ribs. And thanks to my brother Tom, I have the best recipe for bringing them to the table perfectly done, with no toughness at all.

The mistake most folks make in doing ribs is to simply slather them with sauce and plop 'em on the grill. They get burned on the outside, underdone on the inside, and tough to boot. Instead, parboil them in advance. Do so by first cutting the slab into separate ribs. Put in a large pot with enough water to cover them, and add the bay leaves, peppercorns, garlic cloves, and vinegar. Bring to a boil, reduce heat, and simmer for 20 minutes. Drain, discard the bay leaves and peppercorns, and pour on your favorite barbecue sauce. Grill just long enough to heat the ribs through, "caramelizing" the barbecue sauce. Enjoy with potato salad and corn on the cob. Ah, life is good!

■ ■ ■ ■ ■ ■ ■ ■ ■ ■ *Short Ribs with Dynamite Sauce*

1 *lb extra-low-fat beef short*
   ribs per person
1 *tbsp canola oil*
½ *cup chopped onion*
1 *15-oz can tomato sauce*
4 *tbsp vinegar*
1 *tbsp ground mustard*
2 *tsp salt*
1 *package brown gravy mix*
   (any brand)
1 *cup red wine*

Brown the short ribs in the canola oil in a dutch oven or other large pot. Drain off oil. Mix all remaining ingredients and pour over the ribs. Bring to a boil, reduce heat, and simmer covered for 1½ to 2 hours until tender and the meat falls off the bone. Serve with noodles or mashed potatoes.

■ ■ ■ ■ ■ ■ ■ ■ ■ ■ ■   *Veal Marsala*

1 *tbsp onion, chopped fine*
1 *tbsp carrot, chopped fine*
1 *tbsp celery leaves, chopped*
   fine
½ *tsp thyme*
1 *bay leaf*
2 *tbsp parsley, minced*
1 *tbsp olive oil*
2 *tbsp flour*
1 *cup beef bouillon*
1 *tbsp tomato paste*
1 *lb veal sliced for scallopini*

There are two options with this classic Italian dish: the no-fuss approach or the more time-consuming perfect version. Option number one, pick up a packet of Lawry's Weekday Gourmet Veal Marsala Sauce. You'll find it along with a number of other Lawry prepared sauces in any super-market. Each packet contains enough for 12 ounces of meat.

Flatten veal cutlets with a kitchen mallet or the flat side of a chef's knife or just use your fist. Sauté in a bit of good olive oil, and then pour the sauce over the meat. Serve with angel hair pasta, which cooks up in just 2 minutes, drizzled with extra-virgin olive oil, and a vegetable.

But if you've got some time, here's the recipe I've grown to love. My wife Dawn discovered it in the *Chicago Sun-Times* two decades ago. Prepare this once, and you'll be hooked.

Sauté onion, carrot, celery leaves, thyme, bay leaf, and parsley in olive oil, about 5 minutes. Sprinkle on and blend in the flour. Add the bouillon and stir frequently over medium heat until the mixture boils and thickens. Stir in the tomato paste and simmer for 5 minutes. Put sauce mixture through a strainer and set aside.

1 cup flour
1 tsp each oregano, thyme,
   salt, pepper
1 tbsp olive oil
8 large mushrooms, sliced
2 large garlic cloves, peeled
   and crushed
1 cup Marsala wine
1 tsp grated parmesan cheese
2 tbsp Italian parsley,
   minced, for garnish
   (regular parsley will do)

Combine the flour and herbs, then dredge the veal slices. Sauté veal in olive oil, about 2 minutes per side. Don't worry about browning it. Remove veal. Add a bit more olive oil to the pan if necessary, and sauté mushrooms and garlic until garlic is tender. Stir in the reserved sauce till warmed, then add the Marsala. Return the veal to the pan and heat through and serve. It's worth the effort! Serve with angel hair pasta and green peas, along with a fine bottle of Italian red wine.

■ ■ ■ ■ ■ ■ ■ ■ ■ ■ ■

Poached Salmon with Green Sauce

2 salmon steaks, about 8 oz
   each
½ lemon, sliced thin

Court Bouillon

1 quart water
1 tbsp fresh lemon juice
2 small carrots, sliced thin
1 small onion, sliced thin
2 bay leaves
6 black peppercorns
1 tsp salt

Green Sauce

¼ cup nonfat sour cream
1½ tbsp low-fat mayo
¼ tsp salt
½ tsp vinegar
1 green onion, chopped fine
5 tbsp fresh dill, chopped
   with stems removed
parsley and lemon slices for
   garnish

I'm a lucky guy. I happen to absolutely love one of the most heart-healthy foods. Salmon drips with omega-3 fatty acids, and I try to find the fattest fish I can. It's great over the coals on the outdoor barbecue, but here's an unusual recipe that's terrific for a romantic evening for two.

One can poach salmon in plain water, but using what's called a *court bouillon* adds a lot of pizzazz. Place all *court bouillon* ingredients in a shallow, flameproof casserole dish and heat on stove top to boiling. Reduce heat and simmer 10 minutes. Place salmon in casserole and spoon ingredients over the steaks and top with slice lemon. Cover with a piece of waxed paper and bake 20 minutes in a 350°F oven.

While salmon is poaching, prepare green sauce. Place all ingredients in a blender and blend at high until smooth.

Serve salmon topped with the green sauce, garnished with parsley and lemon slices. Rice and asparagus go well with this dish. And, of course, a chilled bottle of white wine.

■ ■ ■ ■ ■ ■ ■ ■ ■ ■ ■ ■ ■ **Blackened Cajun Salmon**

4 *8-oz salmon fillets*
2 *tbsp tub or squeeze-bottle margarine*

Cajun Blackening Seasoning

1 *tbsp paprika*
1 *tsp garlic powder*
1 *tsp cayenne*
³⁄₄ *tsp ground black pepper*
¹⁄₂ *tsp ground thyme*
¹⁄₂ *tsp oregano*
¹⁄₂ *tsp dried basil*
1 *tsp onion powder*
2 *tsp salt*

*Place skillet directly on hot coals in the outdoor barbecue grill. Allow to heat until white hot. When you put the fish on the skillet, there will be a huge cloud of smoke. Ross used to get a big kick out of that when he was a kid. In fact, both of us still do!

Few chefs leave such a signature dish as Paul Prudhomme has with blackened fish. If you've enjoyed this dish in restaurants, why not try making it at home. It's really a lot of fun, but because of the smoke produced, you'll need to do it outside unless you have a very powerful exhaust fan over the stove.* You can buy blackening seasonings, but you'll save a lot of money by making your own. Double or triple the recipe for future use.

Mix all the seasonings together. Sprinkle liberally over salmon fillets. Place seasoned fillets with ¹⁄₂ tbsp of margarine each in a *very* hot cast-iron skillet. Sear for 2 minutes, then turn and blacken for another 2 minutes. This is a spicy dish and goes best with a cold glass of beer. Serve with rice and carrots.

■ ■ ■ ■ ■ ■ ■ ■ ■ ■ ■ *Linguini and*
White Clam Sauce

1 *6.5-oz can chopped clams*
2 *tbsp extra-virgin olive oil*
2 *cloves garlic, minced*
¼ *cup onion, minced*
½ *cup white wine*
½ *pound linguini*
water
¼ *cup parsley, chopped fine*

This truly elegant dish can be
thrown together in just a few
minutes. It's so simple that I got it
in conversation with a cardiologist
as we were having dinner. I'll
bet you pass it on to your friends
as well.

Linguini takes 12 minutes to cook, so begin by cooking it according to directions on the package in salted water. In the time it takes to cook the pasta, your clam sauce will be ready. Drain clams and reserve liquid. Heat olive oil in skillet and sauté clams, garlic, and onion until the onion is transparent, about 4 minutes. Add white wine and clam liquid, bring to a boil, reduce heat, and simmer until pasta is ready, thus reducing total. Add parsley and heat through. Drain linguini, serve with clam sauce. Enjoy with the rest of the bottle of white wine and a crusty loaf of bread and a side salad.

■ ■ ■ ■ ■ ■ ■ ■ ■ ■ ■ *New England Clam Chowder*

1 *6.5-oz can minced clams*
1 *6.5-oz can whole clams*
2 *tbsp olive oil*
½ *cup onion, chopped*
2 *cups potatoes, peeled and*
   cubed
1 *14.5-oz can low-sodium*
   chicken broth
½ *tsp freshly ground pepper*
½ *cup Land o' Lakes fat-free*
   half-and-half

When clam chowder's on a
restaurant menu I always ask if it's
the Manhattan (red) or New
England (white) version. I have
to turn down the latter, since it's
made with butter and cream. No
big deal, there are always other
options available. And I can
have my creamy New England
chowder at home with this
recipe.

Drain clams, reserve liquid. Heat olive oil in saucepan large enough to accommodate all ingredients. Sauté clams and onion until onion is transparent. Add potatoes and chicken broth. Cook until potatoes are tender. Season with salt and pepper. Stir in half-and-half. Serve with oyster crackers.

■ ■ ■ ■ ■ ■ ■ ■ ■ ■ ■

Skewering Ingredients

1 *pound assorted seafood: shrimp, large sea scallops, fish*

Marinade

½ *cup chicken broth*
1 *tbsp each lime, lemon, and orange juice and cider vinegar*
2 *tbsp canola oil*
3 *tbsp finely chopped parsley*
3 *cloves garlic, minced*
½ *tsp each salt and white pepper*

Shrimp 'n' Scallops on the Barby

You can use this recipe with any fish or seafood combination you wish. It doesn't call for vegetables, but if you want to skewer some veggies just double the marinade ingredients. But cook the veggies separately, since they take longer to cook than either shrimp or scallops.

Peel and devein shrimp. Rinse scallops. Cut fish into chunks. Mix the marinade ingredients in a large plastic food storage bag. Place seafood in bag and refrigerate 2 to 3 hours. Skewer the seafood alternately, and broil or grill until shrimp and scallops lose their translucency; do not overcook these delicate foods. *Serves 4.*

■ ■ ■ ■ ■ ■ ■ ■ ■ ■ ■ ■

Herbed Pork and Vegetable Skewers

This truly is a meal on a skewer. No need for muss and fuss at the picnic site. Be sure not to overcook the pork.

Marinade

- 1 cup beef broth
- 2 tbsp lime juice
- 2 tbsp canola oil
- 1 tsp each oregano, thyme, onion powder, sage
- 4 cloves garlic, minced

Skewering Ingredients

- 1 lb pork tenderloin, trimmed and cut in cubes
- 1 lb small potatoes (red or yellow)
- 1 lb large mushrooms, ends trimmed
- 2 bell peppers, cut in eighths (green or mix colors)
- 2 onions, cut in quarters

Mix the marinade ingredients together in a large plastic food storage bag. Prepare the meat and vegetables and put in with marinade for 2 to 3 hours in the refrigerator. Skewer the meat and vegetables alternately and cook over coals until vegetables are tender and pork is barely pink. Serves 4.

■ ■ ■ ■ ■ ■ ■ ■ ■ ■ ■ ■ *Shepherd's Pie*

1 tbsp canola oil
1 lb low-fat ground beef
½ cup chopped onions
1 tbsp paprika
1 tsp onion powder
1 tsp garlic powder
1 tsp white pepper
1 tsp salt
1 bay leaf
4 oz water
1 16-oz package frozen peas
  and carrots
mashed potatoes (see page 237)

When they were traveling in Australia with me while I was on a media tour for one of my books, my family fell in love with what was originally a British dish called shepherd's pie. This is a mixture of minced lamb with peas and carrots, topped with mashed potatoes as the "crust" and baked. Of course, as served in the restaurant, that Aussi pie was extremely high in fat. So I came up with a healthier version.

Heat canola oil in a skillet, then brown ground beef until crumbly. Add remaining ingredients except potatoes. Bring to a bubble and simmer for 5 minutes. Spray a 9 × 9-inch casserole dish with vegetable spray. Spread meat mixture, mixed with the peas and carrots, in the casserole dish and top with plenty of mashed potatoes to form a crust 1 to 2 inches thick. Bake in a preheated 400°F oven for 30 minutes.

Here's an opportunity to make another meal in advance. Do 2 pies. Bake 1 for that evening, and freeze the other for one of those hectic evenings.

Serve with a salad, if you'd like, and some crusty bread. G'day, mate!

■ ■ ■ ■ ■ ■ ■ ■ ■ ■ ■ ■ *Thai Chicken with*
Peanut Sauce

4 6-oz skinless chicken
   breasts
2 tbsp smooth-style peanut
   butter
2 tbsp each soy sauce and
   sake
1 tbsp brown sugar
3 cloves garlic, chopped fine
2 tsp fresh lime juice
½ tsp red pepper flakes
¼ cup cilantro, chopped,
   without stems

*Chicken and turkey got a lot of
attention in my first book, in the
days when red meat was limited.
Ironically, this recipe wouldn't
have made the cut back then
because peanut butter is high in fat.
But today we know that this
monounsaturated fat has no effect
on cholesterol levels.*

Broil the chicken breasts. Blend
peanut butter with soy sauce and
sake until smooth. If you don't
have sake, you can substitute rice
vinegar or even water. Add
remaining ingredients and mix.
Serve over broiled chicken breasts
with rice and asparagus.

■ ■ ■ ■ ■ ■ ■ ■ ■ ■ ■ ■ *Breakfast and Pizza Sausage*

*In the many years of my writing my
books and newsletter, companies
come and companies go. It's nice to
see a good one stand the test of
time. Spice 'n' Slice sausage mixes
allow you to make your own fresh,
low-fat sausage at home.*

Call to place an order for the
sausage mixes from Spice 'n' Slice
at 800-310-4094. Keep several
packets on hand in your pantry.
The sealed packets last indefinitely.
Ask about their variety of spice
and seasonings packets.

The company makes a wide
variety of flavors for pepperoni,
salami, bologna, and others.

Hunters rely on the mixes to produce sausage from the wild game they bring home. My own favorites are the breakfast sausage mixes, in Southern (spicy) and Country Style flavors.

For *breakfast sausage*, just mix the contents of the packet with 2 lbs of ground pork. To get the lowest fat, of course, have your butcher trim off the fat and grind a chunk of pork loin or tenderloin. Form 2-oz or 3-oz patties, use whatever you need at the time, and freeze the rest for future use.

Breakfast pork sausage is not only for breakfast in our house. Again, this is a midwestern taste, but we like to have a couple of patties along with mashed potatoes and pork gravy with some applesauce. Peas and carrots seem to go particularly well with this easy-to-prepare meal.

For *pizza sausage*, start with the Southern (spicy) breakfast sausage mix and add 1 tbsp of crushed fennel seeds. Mix it all in with 2 lbs of lean ground beef. Again, use what you need for that evening's pizza, and freeze the rest in 4-oz balls, individually plastic-wrapped, for the future. The pizza sausage is also delicious blended into spaghetti sauce, or pan-fried in some olive oil along with pasta and sauce.

■ ■ ■ ■ ■ ■ ■ ■ ■ ■ ■ *Pizza*

There's nothing easier than making your own pizzas at home. Once you do your first one, you'll see no need to ever order the high-sat-fat varieties—and you'll save a lot of money in the bargain.

Simply start with a premade pizza crust. I get mine at the local Italian deli. You can also find frozen pizza crusts in some supermarkets. And you can use frozen and thawed bread dough rolled out into a square or circular crust.

Spread the crust with any commercially prepared pizza sauce. Top with shredded low-fat mozzarella cheese. Sargento and Healthy Choice are good brands. Next, pile on the bits of pizza sausage. I also like to finely chop a bell pepper or two, perhaps a red one and a green one, and put that on as well. Serve with a salad and you've got a complete, balanced, low-fat meal. Preheat the oven to 400°F and bake on a large cookie pan or a specially designed pizza pan for 10 to 15 minutes, depending on how much topping you've used. Delicious with a glass of nice Italian red wine!

THE DIET-HEART NEWSLETTER

Since *The 8-Week Cholesterol Cure* was published in 1987, I've been keeping my readers up to date on the latest developments in heart health by way of my quarterly publication, *The Diet-Heart Newsletter*.

Each issue brings updates on scientific and medical research, new foods and heart-healthy products, insider reports from professional meetings, and answers to readers' questions. It's my continuing link with you.

To receive a sample issue and subscription information, please send a self-addressed, stamped, business-size envelope to:

The Diet-Heart Newsletter
PO Box 2039
Venice, CA 90294

References

Chapter 1: Way Beyond Cholesterol

CHOLESTEROL

Andrews, TC, et al. Effect of cholesterol reduction on myocardial ischemia in patients with coronary disease. *Circulation.* January 1997.

Danesh, J, et al. Lipoprotein(a) and risk of myocardial infarction. *Circulation.* September 2000.

Dansky, HM, and Fisher, EA. High-density lipoprotein and plaque regression: the good cholesterol gets even better. *Circulation.* November 1999.

Dupuis, J, et al. Cholesterol reduction rapidly improves endothelial function after acute coronary syndromes. *Circulation.* June 1999.

Enas, EA. Triglycerides and small, dense low-density lipoprotein. *Journal of the American Medical Association.* December 1998.

Forrester, JS, and Prediman, KS. Lipid lowering versus revascularization. *Circulation.* August 1997.

Frye, RL. Clinical reality of lowering total and LDL cholesterol. *Circulation.* January 1997.

Goldbourt, U, et al. High HDL cholesterol lowers stroke risk. *Stroke.* January 1997.

Gotto, AM. Low high-density lipoprotein cholesterol as a risk factor in coronary heart disease: a working group report. *Circulation.* May 2001.

Hodis, HN, et al. Intermediate-density lipoproteins and progression of carotid arterial wall intima-media thickness. *Circulation.* April 1997.

Huggins, GS, et al. Effects of short-term treatment of hyperlipidemia on coronary vasodilator function and myocardial perfusion in regions having substantial impairment of baseline dilator reserve. *Circulation.* September 1998.

Lamarche, B, et al. Small, dense low-density lipoprotein particles as a predictor of the risk of ischemic heart disease in men. *Circulation.* January 1997.

Moroney, JT, et al. Low-density lipoprotein cholesterol and the risk of dementia with stroke. *Journal of the American Medical Association*. July 1999.

O'Hanesian, MA, et al. Effects of inherent responsiveness to diet and day-to-day diet variation on plasma lipoprotein concentrations. *American Journal of Clinical Nutrition*. July 1996.

Pearson, TA, et al. Most patients do not achieve target LDL cholesterol levels. *Archives of Internal Medicine*. February 2000.

Schaefer, EJ, et al. Lipoprotein (a) levels and risk of coronary heart disease in men. *Journal of the American Medical Association*. April 1994.

Stone, NJ, et al. Summary of the scientific conference on the efficacy of hypocholesterolemic dietary interventions. *Circulation*. December 1996.

Superko, HR. Beyond LDL cholesterol reduction. *Circulation*. November 1996.

Vakkailainen, J, et al. Endothelial dysfunction in men with small LDL particles. *Circulation*. August 2000.

SCREENING FOR CALCIUM: EBCT

Achenbach, S, et al. Value of electron-beam computed tomography for the noninvasive detection of high-grade coronary-artery stenoses and occlusions. *New England Journal of Medicine*. December 1999.

Callister, TQ, et al. Effect of HMG-coA reductase inhibitors on coronary artery disease as assessed by electron-beam tomography. *New England Journal of Medicine*. December 1999.

Rumberger, JA. Electron beam (ultrafast) computed tomography for the evaluation of cardiac disease and function. *Medscape* (www.medscape.com). November 17, 2000.

Lp(a)

Rader, DJ, and Brewer, HB. Lipoprotein (a): Clinical approach to a unique atherogenic lipoprotein. *Journal of the American Medical Association*. February 1992.

Ridker, PM, et al. Plasma concentration of lipoprotein (a) and the risk of future stroke. *Journal of the American Medical Association*. April 1995.

URIC ACID

Fang, J, and Alderman, MH. Serum uric acid and cardiovascular mortality. *Journal of the American Medical Association*. May 2000.

GLUCOSE

Wei, M, et al. Low fasting plasma glucose level as a predictor of cardiovascular disease and all-cause mortality. *Circulation*. May 2000.

DIABETES AND HEART DISEASE

Despres, JP, et al. Hyperinsulinemia as an independent risk factor for ischemic heart disease. *New England Journal of Medicine.* April 1996.

Reaven, GM. Insulin resistance, its consequences, and coronary heart disease. *Circulation.* May 1996.

Steinberg, HO, et al. Type II diabetes abrogates sex differences in endothelial function in premenopausal women. *Circulation.* May 2000.

IRON

Ascherio, A, and Willet, WC. Are body iron stores related to the risk of coronary heart disease? *New England Journal of Medicine.* August 1994.

Danesh, J, and Appleby, P. Coronary heart disease and iron status. *Circulation.* February 1999.

Duffy, SJ, et al. Iron chelation improves endothelial function in patients with coronary artery disease. *Circulation.* June 2001.

Mann, D. Blood donation may decrease MI risk by lowering iron levels. *Medical Tribune.* April 1997.

Matsuoka, H, et al. High iron levels may speed atherosclerosis. *American Heart Association Advisory.* October 2000.

HOMOCYSTEINE

Anderson, JL, et al. Plasma homocysteine predicts mortality independently of traditional risk factors. *Circulation.* September 2000.

Boushey, CJ, et al. A quantitative assessment of plasma homocysteine as a risk factor for vascular disease. *Journal of the American Medical Association.* October 1995.

Friso, S, et al. Low circulating vitamin B_6 is associated with elevation of the inflammation marker C-reactive protein independently of plasma homocysteine levels. *Circulation.* June 2001.

Omenn, GS, et al. Preventing coronary heart disease: B vitamins and homocysteine. *Circulation.* January 1998.

Ridker, PM, et al. Homocysteine and risk of cardiovascular disease among postmenopausal women. *Journal of the American Medical Association.* May 1999.

Scott, JM. Homocysteine and cardiovascular risk. *American Journal of Clinical Nutrition.* August 2000.

BLOOD CLOTS

American Heart Association. Physicians urged to measure fibrinogen, a clotting protein linked to "very bad" LDL. January 1996.

Danesh, J, et al. Association of fibrinogen with coronary heart disease. *Journal of the American Medical Association.* May 1998.

Montalescot, G, et al. Fibrinogen after coronary angioplasty as a risk factor for restenosis. *Circulation.* July 1995.

INFLAMMATION

Danesh, J, et al. Low-grade inflammation and coronary heart disease. *British Medical Journal.* July 2000.

Gussekloo, J, et al. C-reactive protein, stroke, and cardiovascular disease. *Arteriosclerosis, Thrombosis, and Vascular Biology.* April 2000.

Lagrand, WK, et al. C-reactive protein as a cardiovascular risk factor. *Circulation.* July 1999.

Oberman, A. Emerging cardiovascular risk factors. *Clinical Reviews.* Spring 2000.

Rader, DJ. Inflammatory markers of coronary risk. *New England Journal of Medicine.* October 2000.

Ridker, PM. High-sensitivity C-reactive protein: Potential adjunct for global risk assessment in the primary prevention of cardiovascular disease. *Circulation.* April 2001.

Ridker, PM, et al. C-reactive protein and other markers of inflammation in the prediction of cardiovascular disease in women. *New England Journal of Medicine.* March 2000.

Tataru, M-C, et al. C-reactive protein concentrations correlate with the severity of atherosclerosis. *European Heart Journal.* June 2000.

GERM THEORY

Folsom, AR. Antibiotics for prevention of myocardial infarction? Not yet! *Journal of the American Medical Association.* February 1999.

Grayston, JT. Antibiotic treatment of *Chlamydia pneumoniae* for secondary prevention of cardiovascular events. *Circulation.* May 1998.

Koenig, W, et al. Infection with *Helicobacter pylori* is not a major independent risk factor for stable coronary heart disease. *Circulation.* December 1999.

Mublestein, JB, et al. Increased incidence of *Chlamydia* species within the coronary arteries of patients with asymptomatic atherosclerotic versus other forms of cardiovascular disease. *Journal of the American College of Cardiology.* June 1996.

Nieto, FJ, et al. Cohort study of cytomegalovirus infection as a risk factor for carotid intimal-medial thickening, a measure of subclinical atherosclerosis. *Circulation.* September 1996.

BLOCKING CHOLESTEROL

Maki, KC, et al. Lipid responses to plant-sterol-enriched reduced-fat spreads incorporated into a National Cholesterol Education Program Step 1 diet. *American Journal of Clinical Nutrition.* July 2001.

Chapter 2: Special Considerations for Women, the Young, and the Elderly

WOMEN

Akahoshi, M, et al. Effects of menopause on trends of serum cholesterol, blood pressure, and body mass index. *Circulation.* July 1996.

Grodstein, F, et al. Postmenopausal estrogen and progestin use and the risk of cardiovascular disease. *New England Journal of Medicine.* August 1996.

Kushi, LH, et al. Physical activity and mortality in postmenopausal women. *Journal of the American Medical Association.* April 1997.

Schrott, HL, et al. Adherence to National Cholesterol Education Program treatment goals in postmenopausal women with heart disease. *Journal of the American Medical Association.* April 1997.

Stampfer, MJ, et al. Primary prevention of coronary disease in women through diet and lifestyle. *New England Journal of Medicine.* July 2000.

THE YOUNG

McGill, HC, et al. Risk factors for heart disease in youth. *Circulation.* July 2000.

National Cholesterol Education Program. *Report of the Expert Panel on Blood Cholesterol Levels in Children and Adolescents.* Bethesda, Md.: U.S. Department of Health and Human Services, Public Health Service, National Institutes of Health, National Heart, Lung, and Blood Institute. 1991. NIH publication 91-2732.

Newman, WP III, et al. Relation of serum lipoprotein levels and systolic blood pressure to early atherosclerosis: The Bogalusa Heart Study. *New England Journal of Medicine.* May 1986.

Niinkoski, H, et al. Prospective randomized trial of low-saturated-fat, low-cholesterol diet during the first 3 years of life. *Circulation.* September 1996.

Rifkind, BM, et al. When should patients with heterozygous familial hypercholesterolemia be treated? *Journal of the American Medical Association.* January 1999.

Stamler, J, et al. Relationship of baseline serum cholesterol levels in 3 large cohorts of younger men to long-term coronary, cardiovascular, and all-cause mortality and to longevity. *Journal of the American Medical Association.* July 2000.

Strong, JP, et al. Prevalence and extent of atherosclerosis in adolescents and young adults. *Journal of the American Medical Association.* February 1999.

THE ELDERLY

Abbott, RD, et al. Walking cuts risk of heart attack in elderly men. *Circulation.* July 1999.

Corti, M-C, et al. Risk of cholesterol and coronary heart disease in the elderly. *Journal of the American Medical Association.* September 1995.

Frost, PH, et al. Coronary heart disease risk factors in men and women aged 60 years and older. *Circulation.* July 1996.

Taddei, S, et al. Physical activity prevents age-related impairment in nitric oxide availability in elderly athletes. *Circulation.* June 2000.

Chapter 4: Good Food, Good Times, Good Health

MOM WAS RIGHT: EAT YOUR FRUITS AND VEGETABLES

Appel, LJ, et al. A clinical trial on the effects of dietary patterns on blood pressure. *New England Journal of Medicine.* April 1997.

Hu, FB, et al. Prospective study of major dietary patterns and risk of coronary heart disease in men. *American Journal of Clinical Nutrition.* October 2000.

Jacobs, DR, et al. It's more than an apple a day: An appropriately processed plant-centered dietary pattern may be good for your health. *American Journal of Clinical Nutrition.* October 2000.

Joshipura, KJ, et al. Fruit and vegetable intake in relation to risk of ischemic stroke. *Journal of the American Medical Association.* October 1999.

Kant, AK. Consumption of energy-dense, nutrient-poor foods by adult Americans. *American Journal of Clinical Nutrition.* October 2000.

Liu, S, et al. Fruit and vegetable intake and risk of cardiovascular disease. *American Journal of Clinical Nutrition.* October 2000.

Rimm, EB, et al. Vegetable, fruit, and cereal fiber intake and risk of coronary heart disease among men. *Journal of the American Medical Association.* February 1996.

FATS: THE GOOD, THE BAD, AND THE UGLY

Albert, CM, et al. Fish consumption and risk of sudden cardiac death. *Journal of the American Medical Association.* January 1998.

Almario, RU, et al. Effects of walnut consumption on plasma fatty acids and lipoproteins in combined hyperlipidemia. *American Journal of Clinical Nutrition.* July 2001.

American Medical Association. Revised dietary guidelines. *Circulation.* October 2000.

Daviglus, ML, et al. Fish consumption and the 30-year risk of fatal myocardial infarction. *New England Journal of Medicine.* April 1997.

Dreon, DM, et al. A very-low-fat diet is not associated with improved lipoprotein profiles in men. *American Journal of Clinical Nutrition.* March 1999.

Dubois, C, et al. Effects of graded amounts of dietary fat on postprandial lipemia and lipoproteins in normolipidemic adults. *American Journal of Clinical Nutrition.* January 1998.

Knopp, RH, et al. Long-term cholesterol-reducing effects of 4 fat-restricted diets in hypercholesterolemic and combined hyperlipidemic men. *Journal of the American Medical Association.* November 1997.

Kris-Etherton, PM, et al. High monounsaturated fatty acid diets lower both plasma cholesterol and triacylglyceral concentrations. *American Journal of Clinical Nutrition.* December 1999.

Lorgeril, M, et al. Mediterranean diet, traditional risk factors, and the rate of cardiovascular complications after myocardial infarction. *Circulation.* February 1999.

Matheson, B, et al. Effect on serum lipids of monounsaturated oils and margarine in the diet of an Antarctic expedition. *American Journal of Clinical Nutrition.* October 1996.

LISTENING TO YOUR INNER CARNIVORE

Albert, CM, et al. Fish consumption and risk of sudden cardiac death. *Journal of the American Medical Association.* January 1998.

American Heart Association. Revised dietary guidelines. *Circulation.* October 2000.

Daviglus, ML, et al. Fish consumption and the 30-year risk of fatal myocardial infarction. *New England Journal of Medicine.* April 1997.

Eaton, SB, et al. *The Paleolithic Prescription.* New York: Harper & Row, 1988.

Mori, TA, et al. Purified eicosapentaenoic and docosahexanoic acids have differential effects on serum lipids. *American Journal of Clinical Nutrition.* July 2000.

Scott, LW, et al. Effects of beef and chicken consumption on plasma lipid levels in hypercholeterolemic men. *Archives of Internal Medicine.* June 1994.

Stark, KD, et al. Effect of a fish-oil concentrate on serum lipids in postmenopausal women. *American Journal of Clinical Nutrition.* August 2000.

GARLIC: WILL A CLOVE A DAY KEEP THE DOCTOR AWAY?

Berthold, HK, et al. Effect of a garlic oil preparation on serum lipoproteins and cholesterol metabolism. *Journal of the American Medical Association.* June 1998.

Isaacson, JL, et al. Garlic powder and plasma lipids and lipoproteins. *Archives of Internal Medicine.* May 1998.

Jain, AK, et al. Can garlic reduce levels of serum lipids? *American Journal of Medicine.* June 1993.

Steiner, M, et al. A double-blind crossover study in moderately hypercholesterolemic men that compared the effect of aged garlic extract and placebo administration on blood lipids. *American Journal of Clinical Nutrition.* November 1996.

LIFTING A GLASS TO HEART HEALTH

Bobak, M, et al. Moderate beer drinking reduces risk of nonfatal MI in men. *British Medical Journal*. May 2000.

Cooper, HA, et al. Light-to-moderate alcohol intake may benefit some heart failure patients. *Journal of the American College of Cardiology*. May 2000.

Lochner, R, et al. Ethanol suppresses smooth muscle cell proliferation in the postprandial state: A new antiatherosclerotic mechanism of ethanol? *American Journal of Clinical Nutrition*. February 1998.

Rimm, EB, et al. Moderate alcohol intake and lower risk of coronary heart disease. *British Medical Journal*. February 1999.

Sacco, RL, et al. The protective effect of moderate alcohol consumption on ischemic stroke. *Journal of the American Medical Association*. January 1999.

Chapter 5: Antioxidants, Supplements, and Your Heart

Campbell, D, et al. Selenium and vitamin E status. *British Journal of Nutrition*. March 1989.

Food & Nutrition Research Briefs. Can antioxidant foods forestall aging? U.S. Department of Agriculture/Agricultural Research Service. April 1999.

Harvard Heart Letter. Vitamin E supplements: To E or not to E? Harvard University Medical School. August 1997.

Heitzer, T, et al. Antioxidant vitamin C has beneficial effect on artery lining. *Circulation*. July 1996.

Kinlay, S, et al. Plasma alpha-tocopherol and coronary endothelium-dependent vasodilator function. *Circulation*. July 1999.

Losonczy, K, et al. Vitamin E and vitamin C supplement use and risk of all-cause and coronary heart disease mortality in older persons. *American Journal of Clinical Nutrition*. August 1996.

Meydani, SN, et al. Vitamin E supplementation and in vivo immune response in healthy elderly subjects. *Journal of the American Medical Association*. May 1997.

Plotnick, GD, et al. Effect of antioxidant vitamins on the transient impairment of endothelium-dependent brachial artery vasoactivity following a single high-fat meal. *Journal of the American Medical Association*. November 1997.

Taddei, S, et al. Vitamin C improves endothelium-dependent vasodilation. *Circulation*. June 1998.

Vitamin E may prevent narrowing of the arteries. Medscape (www.medscape.com). April 19, 2000.

Chapter 6: Yup, Oat Bran Really Works

Brown, L, et al. Cholesterol-lowering effects of dietary fiber. *American Journal of Clinical Nutrition.* July 1999.

Davidson, MH, et al. Long-term effects of consuming foods containing psyllium seed husk on serum lipids in subjects with hypercholesterolemia. *American Journal of Clinical Nutrition.* May 1999.

Jenkins, DJA, et al. Viscous fibers, health claims, and strategies to reduce cardiovascular disease risk. *American Journal of Clinical Nutrition.* September 2000.

Liu, S, et al. Whole-grain consumption and risk of coronary heart disease: Results from the Nurses' Health Study. *American Journal of Clinical Nutrition.* August 1999.

Nicolosi, R, et al. Plasma lipid changes after supplementation with beta-glucan fiber. *American Journal of Clinical Nutrition.* August 1999.

Pietinen, P, et al. Intake of dietary fiber and risk of coronary heart disease in a cohort of Finnish men. *Circulation.* December 1996.

Wolk, A, et al. Long-term intake of dietary fiber and decreased risk of coronary heart disease among women. *Journal of the American Medical Association.* June 1999.

Chapter 7: Blocking Cholesterol in the Foods You Love

De Oliveira e Silva, ER, et al. Effects of shrimp consumption on plasma lipoproteins. *American Journal of Clinical Nutrition.* October 1996.

Howard, BV, and Kritchevsky, D. Phytochemicals and cardiovascular disease: A statement for healthcare professionals from the American Heart Association. *Circulation.* June 1997.

Jones, PJH, et al. Cholesterol-lowering efficacy of a sitostanol-containing phytosterol mixture with a prudent diet in hyperlipidemic men. *American Journal of Clinical Nutrition.* March 1999.

Mattson, FH, et al. Optimizing the effect of plant sterols on cholesterol absorption in man. *American Journal of Clinical Nutrition.* April 1982.

Miettinen, TA, et al. Reduction of serum cholesterol with sitostanol-ester margarine in a mildly hypercholesterolemic population. *New England Journal of Medicine.* November 1995.

Normen, L, et al. Soy sterol esters and beta-sitostanol ester as inhibitors of cholesterol absorption in human small bowel. *American Journal of Clinical Nutrition.* October 1999.

Pelletier, X, et al. A diet moderately enriched in phytosterols lowers plasma cholesterol concentrations in normocholesterolemic humans. *Annals of Nutrition and Metabolism.* March 1995.

Vuorio, AF, et al. Special margarine cuts cholesterol levels in children with genetic risk of early heart disease. *Arteriosclerosis, Thrombosis, and Vascular Biology.* February 2000.

Chapter 8: Niacin: Fighting for Your Healthy Heart

Aronov, DM, et al. Clinical trial of wax-matrix sustained-release niacin in a Russian population with hypercholesterolemia. *Archives of Family Medicine.* November–December 1996.

Berge, KG, and Canner, RL. Coronary drug project: Experience with niacin. *European Journal of Clinical Pharmacology* (Supplement). 1991.

Brown, G, et al. Regression of coronary artery disease as a result of intensive lipid-lowering therapy. *New England Journal of Medicine.* May 1990.

Carlson, LA, et al. Pronounced lowering of serum levels of lipoprotein Lp(a) in hyperlipidemic subjects treated with nicotinic acid. *Journal of Internal Medicine.* February 1989.

Elam, MB, et al. Effect of niacin on lipid and lipoprotein levels and glycemic control in patients with diabetes and peripheral arterial disease. *Journal of the American Medical Association.* September 2000.

Keenan, JM, et al. Niacin revisited. A randomized, controlled trial of wax-matrix sustained-release niacin in hypercholesterolemia. *Archives of Internal Medicine.* July 1991.

Pasternak, RC, et al. Effect of combination therapy with lipid-lowering drugs in patients with coronary artery disease and "normal" cholesterol levels. *Annals of Internal Medicine.* October 1996.

Chapter 10: Take Your Heart Out for a Walk

Anderson, RE, et al. Effects of lifestyle activity vs structured aerobic exercise in obese women. *Journal of the American Medical Association.* August 1999.

Blair, SN, et al. Influences of cardiorespiratory fitness and other precursors on cardiovascular disease and all-cause mortality in men and women. *Journal of the American Medical Association.* July 1996.

Koenig, W, et al. Leisure-time activity but not work-related physical activity associated with decreased plasma viscosity. *Circulation.* January 1997.

Lee, CD, et al. Cardiorespiratory fitness, body composition, and all-cause and cardiovascular disease mortality in me. *American Journal of Clinical Nutrition.* March 1999.

Manson, JE, et al. A prospective study of walking as compared with vigorous exercise in the prevention of coronary heart disease in women. *New England Journal of Medicine.* August 1999.

Parkkari, J, et al. A controlled trial of the health benefits of regular walking on a golf course. *American Journal of Medicine.* August 2000.

Sesso, HD, et al. Physical activity and coronary heart disease in men: The Harvard Alumni Health Study. *Circulation.* August 2000.

Chapter 11: Sensible Solutions to Blood Pressure Control

Ascherio, A, et al. Intake of potassium, magnesium, calcium, and fiber and risk of stroke among U.S. men. *Circulation.* September 1998.

Bucher, HC, et al. Effect of calcium supplementation on pregnancy-induced hypertension and preeclampsia. *Journal of the American Medical Association.* April 1996.

Graudal, NA, et al. Effects of sodium restriction on blood pressure. *Journal of the American Medical Association.* May 1998.

Hunt, SC, et al. Salt gene determines benefit of low-salt diet. *Hypertension.* September 1998.

McCarron, DA. The dietary guideline for sodium: Should we shake it up? Yes! *American Journal of Clinical Nutrition.* March 2000.

Modica, P. Home devices accurate in measuring blood pressure. *Medical Tribune.* June 1997.

Chapter 13: The Heart of Your Emotions

Barefoot, JC, et al. Symptoms of depression, acute myocardial infarction, and total mortality in a community sample. *Circulation.* May 1996.

Gullette, ECD, et al. Effects of mental stress on myocardial ischemia during daily life. *Journal of the American Medical Association.* May 1997.

Hippisley-Cox, J, et al. Depression as a risk factor for ischemic heart disease in men. *British Medical Journal.* June 1998.

Jiang, W, et al. Mental stress-induced myocardial ischemia and cardiac events. *Journal of the American Medical Association.* June 1996.

Kawachi, I, et al. A prospective study of anger and coronary heart disease. *Circulation.* October 1996.

Kral, BG, et al. Exaggerated reactivity to mental stress is associated with exercise-induced myocardial ischemia in an asymptomatic high-risk population. *Circulation.* December 1997.

Krantz, DS, et al. Effects of mental stress in patients with coronary artery disease. *Journal of the American Medical Association.* April 2000.

Pratt, LA, et al. Depression, psychotropic medication, and risk of myocardial infarction. *Circulation.* December 1996.

Williams, JE, et al. Anger proneness predicts coronary heart disease risk. *Circulation.* May 2000.

Index